THE
IMMUNITY
FOOD FIX
COOKBOOK

75 nourishing recipes that reverse inflammation, heal the gut, detoxify, and prevent illness

Donna Beydoun Mazzola
PharmD, MBA, MS,
Author of *Immunity Food Fix*

with recipes and photography by
Sarah Steffens

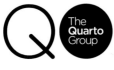

© 2023 Quarto Publishing Group USA Inc.
Text © 2023 Donna Mazzola

First Published in 2023 by Fair Winds Press, an imprint of The Quarto Group,
100 Cummings Center, Suite 265-D, Beverly, MA 01915, USA.
T (978) 282-9590 F (978) 283-2742 Quarto.com

Fair Winds Press titles are also available at discount for retail, wholesale, promotional, and bulk purchase. For details, contact the Special Sales Manager by email at specialsales@quarto.com or by mail at The Quarto Group, Attn: Special Sales Manager, 100 Cummings Center, Suite 265-D, Beverly, MA 01915, USA.

27 26 25 24 23   1 2 3 4 5

ISBN: 978-0-7603-8118-2

Digital edition published in 2023
eISBN: 978-0-7603-8119-9

Library of Congress Cataloging-in-Publication Data available

Design and Page Layout: Stacy Wakefield Forte

Photography: Sarah Steffens

Printed in China

The information in this book is for educational purposes only. It is not intended to replace the advice of a physician or medical practitioner. Please see your health-care provider before beginning any new health program.

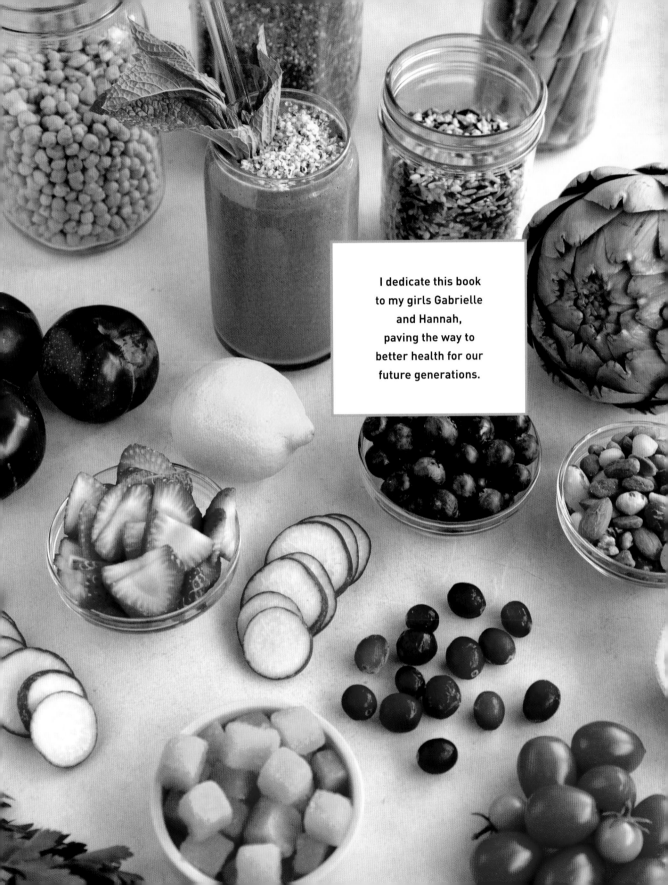

I dedicate this book
to my girls Gabrielle
and Hannah,
paving the way to
better health for our
future generations.

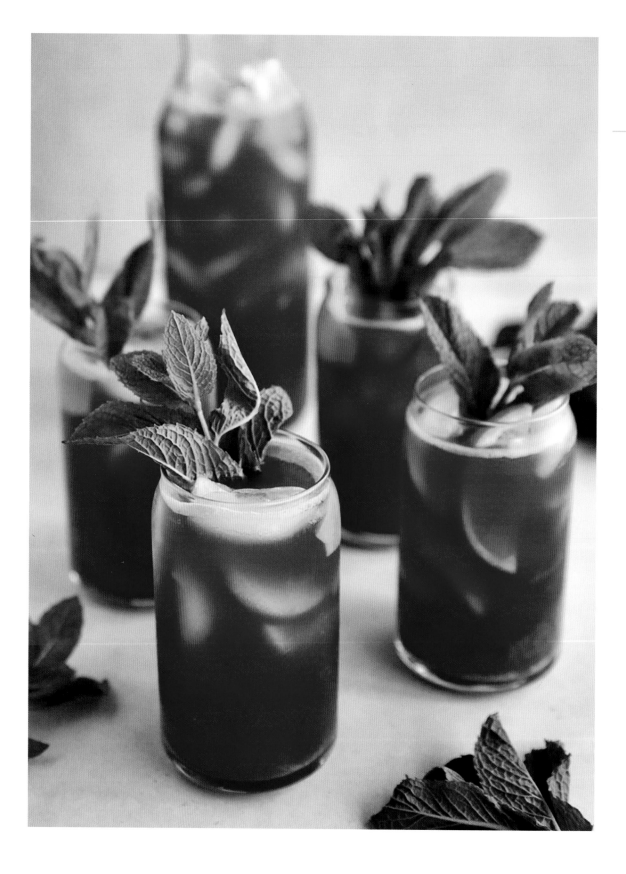

Contents

INTRODUCTION

Food has a powerful impact on the immune system. This can be negative, in the form of serious disease, and it can be powerfully positive, strengthening your overall health and well-being. Today, the majority of the U.S. population lives in a chronic inflammatory state due to the highly processed Western diet. This is leading to the rise in autoimmune disease, as well as increased cardiovascular disease, cognitive decline, and metabolic disorders.

In some ways it's not surprising that this is where so many people are in terms of health and diet. I am a conventionally trained pharmacist, but my education in nutrition was limited. (Unfortunately, it's not part of the medical curriculum.) As I managed my own personal health struggles with autoimmunity, I earned my master's degree in functional medicine and human nutrition, and I did an enormous amount of research to develop my first book, *Immunity Food Fix*. Through this I've come to learn that diet and lifestyle are KEY to reversing and preventing disease.

WHAT YOU EAT MATTERS

In the *Immunity Food Fix* we learned the basics of the immune system and the impact of food on inflammation. This is integral to understanding how powerful the immune system is, both positively and negatively. The science and research around food is plentiful, if not more than the science and research related to medication.

In the *Immunity Food Fix Cookbook* we begin with a deeper dive into how food, immunity, and health are all connected: how food impacts the digestive system, the impact of micronutrients and macronutrients on immunity, and the connection between the immune system and metabolism. My approach is about gaining knowledge, understanding the why behind the process. It's about understanding how the body works and why it "reacts" when given the *wrong* foods or processed foods. It's connecting the dots between the different organ systems and recognizing how they work together to keep us healthy, both our immune health and our metabolic health.

So what do you do with this information? How do you apply it? Where do you start? This book helps you change how you eat in a *balanced* way. There's no need to become obsessive about food and food intake. And there's no reason to suffer through change. As you'll see, you can eat food that tastes amazing *and* is great for your body. The recipes included in this book are packed with anti-inflammatory phytonutrients, antioxidants, micronutrients, and a well-balanced macronutrient

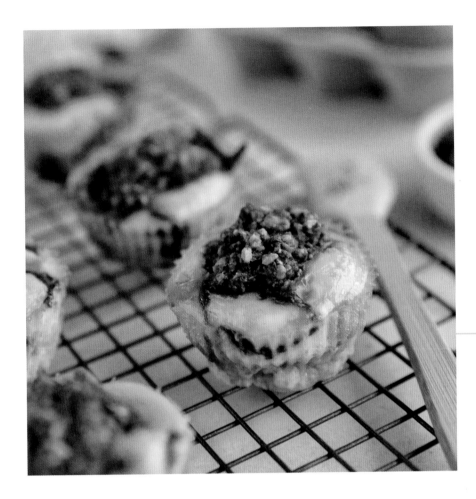

Egg Muffins with
Butternut and
Sunflower Seed
Pesto, page 106

breakdown. There is something in here for every-one. And quite honestly, it's a good place to start, because you have to start somewhere.

Sound like a lot? Don't worry. It doesn't have to be complicated. Just remember this: What we do matters. What we eat matters. How we live matters. I've been living and breathing this lifestyle for more than eight years, and I can't wait for you to dive in. I'm excited to be able to empower you with knowledge about food and your body to make the changes to combat disease and be your best self. Imagine not being fearful of getting sick because you know your body is well supported through the diet you eat. These recipes allow your body to work with you, not against you!

I am confident that this is the perfect tool to build your anti-inflammatory lifestyle, but the bottom line is you have to feel the difference in order to make the change a permanent one. And when you make those changes, you will *feel* what I'm talking about. You will be more energized and less puffy. You will feel refreshed and sleep better. Your body will thank you when you show it care through the food you eat—and once you know what it feels like to be healthy, you will never look back.

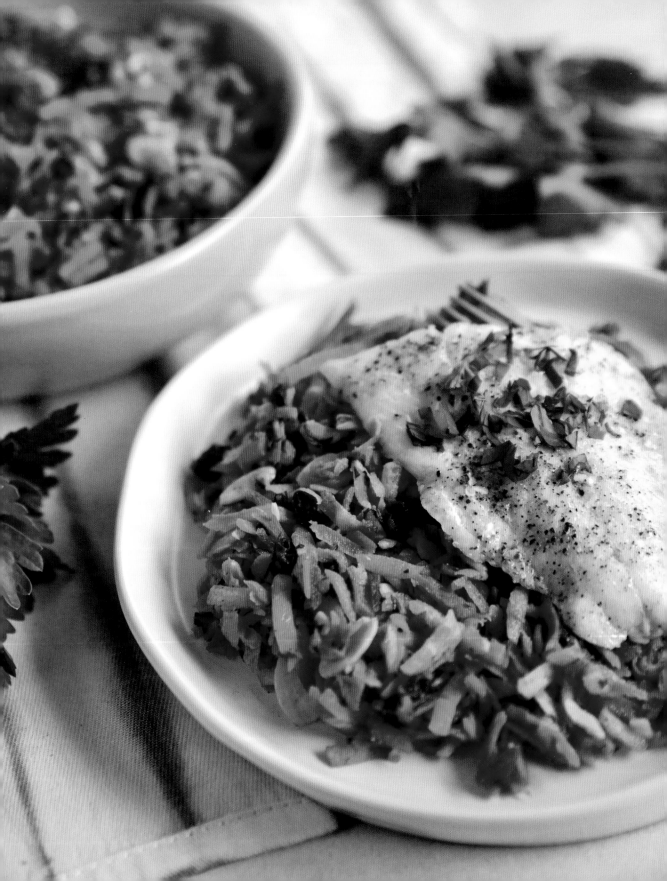

CHAPTER ONE

DIET & THE IMMUNE SYSTEM

In this chapter, we will learn about the connection between intestinal permeability (leaky gut) and gut bacteria. We'll talk about how food impacts gut bacteria and the vicious cycle that can occur when there is an imbalance. We will learn why what we eat matters and how it impacts our gut microbiome and immunity. We also will connect the dots between the multiple organ systems and processes involved in gut homeostasis: the lymphatic system, liver, and bile. What we eat doesn't only matter at a cellular level; it also matters in how our organ systems are connected and how it impacts the entire digestive process.

Moroccan-Spiced Carrot and Parsnip Salad with Lemon-Roasted Cod, page 158

YOUR IMMUNE SYSTEM

The immune system can be broken down into three segments: mucosal, innate, and adaptive. Think of your mucosal immune system as your first line of defense. It's the security checkpoint in areas of your body that interact with the outside world (e.g., skin, mucus, saliva, stomach acid). When a foreign substance gets past this first line, the innate immune system kicks in as a response team to stop an invader or infection. When that isn't enough, the adaptive immune system activates and gives a more specific response.

Your gut is the largest component of your mucosal immune system (mucosal-associated lymphoid tissue). The human gut provides an environment that allows for nutrients to break down and absorption to occur. The gut also forms a mucosal barrier to keep toxins from flowing into the bloodstream. This is a key role in immune defense, and when this process is damaged, problems arise.

There are three key players in your immune system. T cells are critical in recognizing antigens and initiating the immune response. B cells are responsible for antibody (immunoglobin Ig) production. They also have a specific response to an antigen. IgA is a key antibody that plays a critical role in maintaining homeostasis and protecting us from reacting to everything we eat. IgA plays a pivotal role in leaky gut healing and in immune defense.

If our mucosal immune system is damaged—let's say we have insufficient IgA—then we activate our innate and adaptive immune cells. This leads to activation of T cells and B cells, and thus the production of antibodies. Antibodies are specific to the pathogen (the foreign invader the body is attacking). This helps the immune system recognize, attack, and destroy that invader.

five classes of antibodies

» **IgM:** Early stage of immunity (made first), responds to everything.

» **IgD:** We don't know a lot about this one, and it's made spontaneously.

» **IgG:** Found in the blood and can persist for long periods of time. It's the main antibody released to neutralize toxins.

» **IgA:** Our first line of defense. Found in the blood and the mucosal surfaces. It plays an important role in neutralizing food antigens, helping maintain immune tolerance, and preventing the development of food allergies

» **IgE:** Plays a role in protection against parasites. When it's produced as a result of food antigens, you get an IgE-mediated allergy—a *true* allergic response.

THE MICROBIOME

The microbiome regulates the mucosal immune system. It consists of bacteria, viruses, and fungi that work together to create a balance within our gut. Normally, the gut is inhabited by trillions of bacteria that help digest food, produce energy, and make important biological chemicals (such as serotonin and dopamine needed for brain function). Gut bacteria also help detoxify and eliminate toxic exposures.

Gut dysbiosis is one of the physiological conditions that can lead to immune dysregulation, nutrient deficiency, and cellular toxicities. Let's define those terms. Your gut is the long hollow tube that stretches from the tip of your tongue right down to your rectum. Dysbiosis is a state of imbalance among the colonies of microorganisms (bacteria, yeast, viruses, parasites, etc.) within the body.

Gut dysbiosis leads to an inability of the body to absorb nutrients it needs to maintain healthy function. It's associated with a multitude of symptoms, such as abdominal pain, food intolerance, gas, bloating, anxiety, depression, joint pain, and overall immune system dysregulation and disease development. Interestingly, the gut microbiota consists of 1,500 different bacterial species, but each individual gut microbiota is comprised of about 160 different species; this demonstrates how different everyone's gut is.

Gut dysbiosis occurs in your gastrointestinal tract, but the factors that lead to it are all around you. A diet low in fiber/fatty acids, and high in added sugars and preservatives, can alter the environment in the gut, allowing the unfavorable bacteria to dominate. Food allergies can cause inflammation and malabsorption of nutrients. Antibiotics, anti-inflammatories, steroids, and acid blockers can all prevent the digestive system

from doing its job properly. Conditions in the gut environment, such as low acid, pancreatic enzyme insufficiency, slow bowel transit time, and low intestinal IgA (mucosal immunity), can all have negative effects.

Heavy metals and other environmental toxins can damage normal function of the gut and prevent absorption of important nutrients. Alcohol can damage the lining of the gut, allowing toxins to leak into the bloodstream. Stress can cause damage to the intestinal lining, disrupting proper digestive function. And overgrowth of yeast, parasites, and bacteria can prevent proper nutrient absorption.

---

what causes gut dysbiosis?

Many factors can contribute to gut dysbiosis. Here are a few examples:

» **Poor diet**

» **Food allergies**

» **Medications**

» **Dysfunction of the gut environment**

» **Environmental toxins**

» **Alcohol**

» **Stress**

» **Overgrowth of yeast, parasites, and bacteria**

DIET IS KEY

Inflammation is a key contributor to dysregulation. This is why we are so focused on anti-inflammatory foods and functional foods. They promote gut healing, support our immune system, and prevent disease.

The human gut provides an environment that allows nutrients to break down and absorption to occur. It also forms a mucosal barrier to keep toxins from flowing into the bloodstream. This is a key role in immune defense: IgA mediates protection at mucosal surfaces by binding to viruses and bacteria to prevent or inhibit their invasion of epithelial cells. Epithelial cells are cells that come from surfaces of your body, such as your skin, blood vessels, urinary tract, and organs. They are the barrier between the inside and outside of your body.

As human beings, we need to create a relationship with our gut! We provide the habitat for our gut to either **flourish** or deteriorate. It's important to **nourish** our microbiome with the proper nutrients and habitat to maintain that mucosal homeostasis, and thus proper immune response.

The good news is that improving intestinal permeability by *increasing* IgA is critical—and it can be done through the healing powers of food. Cranberries, cherries, papaya, sweet potatoes, and garlic are just a few functional foods we talk about in the *Immunity Food Fix* to boost IgA!

LET'S TALK ABOUT LEAKY GUT

Leaky gut is scientifically known as intestinal permeability. It involves controlling the passage of nutrients and foreign invaders from the gut, through the cells that line the gut, and into the rest of the body.

We have tight junctions (TJs) that seal our gut and prevent outside pathogens from entering and slipping through to our bloodstream. The gut must be porous enough to allow our body to digest food and nutrients while solid enough to carefully regulate this flow and keep out unwanted materials.

Three proteins play key roles in gut health:

» Zonulin modulates leaky gut, and it is upregulated in several autoimmune diseases.

» Occludin holds together the tight junctions of the gut lining.

» Actomyosin maintains the flexibility of the tight junctions of the gut lining.

Under normal conditions, the intestinal wall has cells that are lined up against each other tightly, like bricks on top of each other with no spaces in between, to prevent large material, as in food, from entering the body. When this tight protective barrier is altered or damaged in some way, a gap is formed, allowing harmful substances, such as large undigested food particles, bacteria, and/or viruses (pathogens), to enter the blood. This causes the body, particularly the immune system, to react, leading to inflammation and leaky gut syndrome.

When all things are balanced in your microbiome, the microbiota that live in your intestines regulate and maintain your gut health. Your gut integrity is important, and dysbiosis—imbalance between good and bad bacteria—can disrupt that. When you have an imbalance between the good and the bad, the bad guys overpower and cause major destruction. The pathogenic (bad) bacteria that are hanging out in your intestine can break

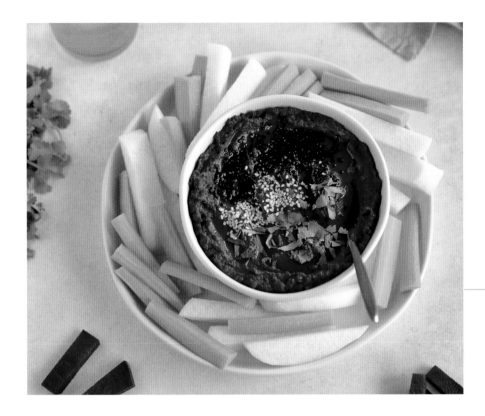

Beet Hummus with Carrot and Jicama Sticks, page 60

down the gut barrier by binding to the epithelial cells or through their ability to release toxins.

LEAKY GUT IN ACTION

To help put this into context, think about a bacterial infection, such as salmonella from food poisoning. The result of that infection is modulation of the intestinal permeability—diarrhea. The diarrhea is not a normal function, but a response to a negative effect because of a known infection.

Now imagine if you eat highly inflammatory foods and avoid anti-inflammatory foods. You will not have proper functioning of your intestinal barrier, and this leads to the "leaking" (translocation) of inflammatory molecules like endotoxins and lipopolysaccharides (LPS) into your bloodstream. This continuous leakage leads to excessive activation of your immune system and a chronic inflammatory response.

What you put in your body impacts your overall well-being. And leaky gut is the biological doorway to an array of diseases, including (but not limited to) irritable bowel syndrome, celiac disease, rheumatoid arthritis, chronic fatigue syndrome, fibromyalgia, allergies, Hashimoto's thyroiditis, and type 1 diabetes.

So, what do you do if you've spent years eating poorly and exposing your gut to all the wrong things? Are you doomed? Of course not! Your gut can rebuild itself, and you can help it! We can influence our microbiota through the foods we eat. In turn, our microbiota will influence the integrity of our gut wall, strengthening our mucosal immune system, preventing disease, and promoting health!

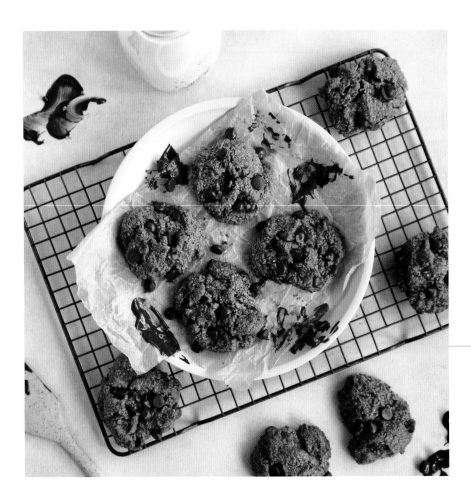

Tahini Chocolate
Chip Cookies,
page 183

OVERNUTRITION AND IMMUNITY

Increased calorie consumption of processed, nutrient-depleted foods impacts your immunity. It's known as the Western diet: the consumption of empty calories from refined grains and sugar and the reliance on animal fat, with no consumption of plant-based, nutrient-dense foods. This overnutrition is what has led to the rise in obesity rates all over the world.

Obesity is connected to inflammatory disease. Evidence suggests that obesity and metabolic disorders are linked to chronic low-grade systemic inflammation. One factor that contributes to this is increased intestinal permeability (leaky gut). In 1995, it was discovered that inflammatory cytokine tumor necrosis factor (TNF)-α levels in fat tissue were increased in obese individuals. Reducing inflammation helps control autoimmune disease and the downstream effect it has on metabolic dysfunction and insulin resistance.

Reducing inflammation isn't easy, but we get it under control by recognizing the root causes. The best place to start is your diet: Is it high in fat? Low in fiber? Fueled by processed sugar? Let's dig in to talk about what happens when we consume a highly inflammatory diet.

HIGH-FAT DIET

Okay, so before you get mad about me saying fat is a bad thing—not all fat is created equal. The amount and type of fats included in the diet influence the degree of inflammation and the risk of chronic disease. Here's what you need to know:

» Anti-inflammatory fats: PUFAs—particularly the long-chain omega-3 fatty acids—*reduce* the risk of heart disease due to their anti-inflammatory potential.

» Inflammatory fats: the increased consumption of saturated fats stimulate inflammatory transcription factor (NF-κβ), resulting in the synthesis of pro-inflammatory cytokines.

What does this mean for your body? An animal study found that feeding mice a high-fat diet for one week impacted the proteins that regulate the tight junctions of the gut wall, leading to permeability and translocation of bacteria into the bloodstream. This also has been identified in humans: Diets high in inflammatory fats correlate to higher levels of LPS in the bloodstream and endotoxemia. That results in leaky gut. It also activates the various cells of the immune system because of this systemic inflammation.

And there's more. High-fat diets can change the composition and diversity of our gut microbiota; we see an increase in proteobacteria and firmicutes and decreased bacteroidetes. Our healthy gut balance is highly dependent on the ratio of firmicutes and bacteroidetes: You want a higher bacteroidetes content than firmicutes to create a balanced environment. An altered F/B ratio alters intestinal permeability and contributes to the pro-inflammatory state. For more details, read about raspberries in the *Immunity Food Fix*.

LOW-FIBER DIET

Dietary fiber supports a healthy gut microbiota, physical barrier function, and immunity. This reduces the risk of developing many of the chronic inflammatory diseases. Low-fiber diets are associated with a low diversity and a pro-inflammatory microbiota.

Dietary fiber is fermented by anaerobic bacteria in the large intestine to produce short-chain fatty acids (SCFAs), which serve as the food for our good bacteria and protect our gut wall. It also reduces the pH in the gut, leading to a more acidic environment, which blocks the bad bacteria from growing. Fiber also has been shown to increase our T regulatory cells and the production of IgA. A lack of SCFA production leads to a reduction in colonic T regulatory cells. Diets high in fruits, vegetables, and whole grains are therefore high in fiber!

SUGARS AND OTHER ADDITIVES

Have you ever thought of the effect of sugar on your gut?! This is complicated, but it's all about balance and the right kind of sugar. Much like fat, not all sugar is created equal. Sugar as glucose is the preferred fuel source for our immune system and proliferation of key components such as TH1 cells, neutrophils, and macrophages. However, when that intake it too high it also increases TH17 cells. TH17 has also been identified as a contributing cause of autoimmune disease. TH1 and TH17 are pro-inflammatory T-helper cells that are associated with the development of autoimmune disorders. Increasing T regulatory cells can help "regulate" or balance these T helper cells, reducing the release of inflammatory cytokines.

Diets high in sucrose can alter digestive enzymes to be able to support processing simple sugars. These enzymes are typically found in anaerobic bacteria and exacerbate intestinal inflammation. If you're eating highly processed foods high in sugar, you're actually changing the composition of your gut bacteria in order to break down all the CRAP, and thus completely changing your gut microbiota.

WHAT A DISRUPTED MICROBIOTA MEANS FOR YOU

So now we have a pretty good understanding of the importance of our gut microbiota and its role in our immune system. Let's take a look at the effects of that disrupted microbiota, specifically the impact on our lymphatic system and key digestive organs.

LEAKY GUT AND THE LYMPHATIC SYSTEM

Think of the lymphatic system as our filtration system's drainpipe. It is responsible for removing fluid, inflammatory cells, and bacterial toxins, and also plays a secondary role in transporting immune cells where needed. It is quite underrated for its role in preventing disease and maintaining health.

When you have leaky gut and dysbiosis in the gut it can significantly impact normal lymphatic function, leading to a clogged drainpipe. This leads to inflammation and disease development. Interestingly, LPS can impact lymph flow rates; if we don't remove those toxins as we should, it can lead to metabolic and inflammatory diseases, as well as weight gain.

LEAKY GUT AND THE LIVER

Think of the liver as the garbage disposal. Everything we eat and consume has to pass through the liver before it can go to the rest of the body or be eliminated. Now think about the amount of toxins you are exposing your body to and the burden that puts on the liver. Chemicals, toxins, pesticides, sugar, alcohol . . . these all increase the toxic load and cause the liver to be more sluggish. The flip side of consuming and exposing ourselves to these toxins is we are not providing the body with the nutrients it needs to function.

The liver receives 70 percent of its blood supply from the large and small intestines through the hepatic portal vein. The various cells of the immune system equip the liver to get rid of toxins; however, leaky gut, which results in translocation of several toxic bacteria, leads to liver (hepatic) inflammation.

A new term buzzing around is nonalcoholic fatty liver disease (NAFLD). NAFLD is associated with an increase in leaky gut, and this is related to the increased prevalence of gut dysbiosis and small intestinal bacterial overgrowth. The gut dysbiosis and translocation of bacteria across the epithelial barrier increases liver dysfunction, leads to NAFLD, and worsens leaky gut. It's a vicious cycle that keeps going around!

BILE ACID

Bile is produced in the liver and stored in the gall-bladder until it is released into the small intestine. There it works to break down fat, which is further broken down by enzymes. When you don't have enough bile salt, you can suffer from gas, bloating, and diarrhea. Bacterial overgrowth disrupts the cells of bile salts; this appears to irritate the mucosal lining of the intestine and causes poor absorption of fatty acids.

Under normal conditions, the consumption of fat results in the release of bile acids. In high-fat diets, the body adapts by increasing bile-tolerant bacteria such as Alistipes, Bilophila, and Bacteroides. So high-fat diets are associated with altered fecal bile acid profiles and increased secondary bile acid metabolites, such as cancer-causing deoxycholic acid (DCA). These organisms are associated with a pro-inflammatory TH1 immune response, increases in hydrogen gas production, and gut inflammation. Ultimately, the level of saturation of dietary fat plays a part in how fecal bile is altered and its contribution to gut inflammation.

Interestingly, bile acids are classified as primary and secondary types. Primary bile acid is released into the intestinal lumen and taken up in the small intestine. About 5 percent of that bile escapes the small intestine and moves into the large intestine. When this happens, the bile acid does a little dance with the bacteria in the gut and produces secondary bile acids. This transformation should occur in 95 percent of the bile acid in an otherwise healthy gut.

If you have dysbiosis, the lack of beneficial bacteria needed to transform the bile acid from primary to secondary is limited, so you get a higher amount of primary bile acid. This is a problem because it increases leaky gut and causes more inflammation in the lining. Just another reason we need an abundance of our Lactobacillus and Bifidobacterium species (good bacteria).

THE ROLE OF THE MICROBIOME

Understanding the role of the microbiome is critical to keeping our immune system balanced and preventing disease. Maintaining our gut barrier is the key. The gut mucosa serves as a barrier, our first line of defense, against foreign antigens. To keep our gut lining healthy, the microbiota that live in our intestinal tract need to be compromised of the good, beneficial bacteria. When we get an overabundance of bad bacteria in the intestine, this increases leaky gut, causing a vicious cycle of inflammation between our digestive organs. Our gut doesn't work in a silo, so we need to connect the dots in how the food we eat is impacting our entire digestive process. Simply put, you can probably relate how you feel to what you eat. Symptoms of gas, bloating, and constipation are not normal after you eat. We need to stop normalizing these symptoms. Remember that what you eat matters, and it's in your hands to nourish your body and feel good doing so.

The good news is you can break this cycle: Avoid foods that lead to intestinal inflammation and leaky gut. Focus on anti-inflammatory, healing foods. The mucosal lining of the gut can be rebuilt. The beneficial bacteria can repopulate. The fix is in the FOOD!

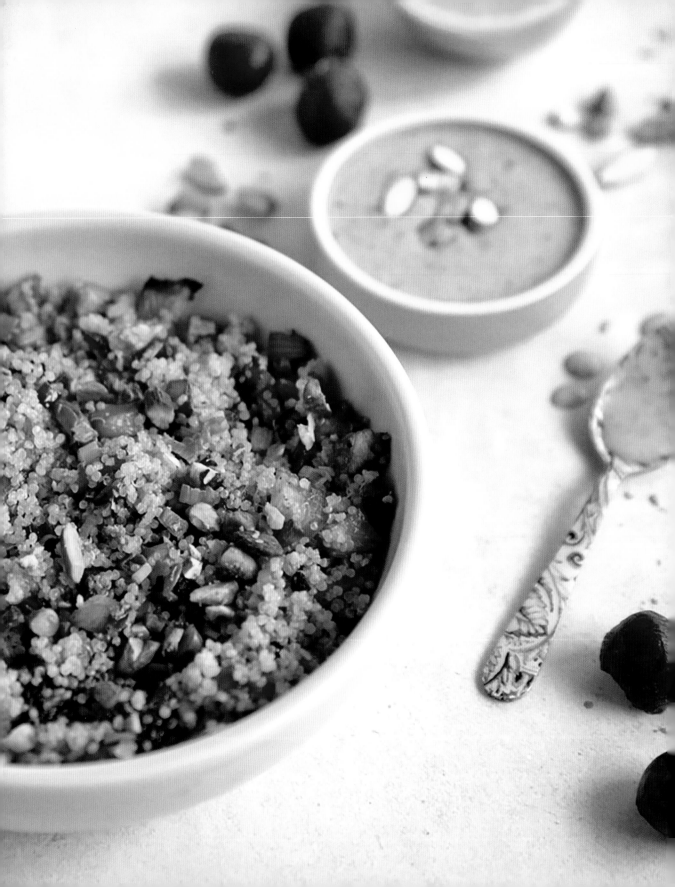

CHAPTER TWO

NUTRITION & IMMUNITY

We know that the microbiome plays a critical role in our body's immune response—but how much does nutrition really matter? A lot! Proper nutrition provides essential support to our immune system. Undernutrition impairs the immune system and suppresses immune function, and overnutrition can lead to excessive inflammation and alter our body's response and function. In this chapter, we will learn about the importance of macronutrients and micronutrients on our immune system, and how they can help us achieve optimal health and prevent disease.

Roasted Cherry and Fennel Quinoa Salad
with Pistachios and Orange-Almond
Dressing, page 154

WHY VITAMINS AND MINERALS MATTER

We often think about vitamins and minerals in relation to an established disease. For instance, calcium and vitamin D are used in response to osteoporosis. Magnesium supplementation is a go-to to ease chronic migraines, and we turn to iron to remedy anemia. Likewise, pharmaceutical medications are used to alter "normal" pathology in an effort to remediate disease.

We also typically follow Dietary Reference Intakes (DRIs): the minimum amounts recommended to prevent an index deficiency disease. To translate this, it's the minimum amount needed to prevent full-on disease. That doesn't mean it's enough. This is different from the variable amount needed for optimal health!

Have you ever thought about vitamins to optimize your health? What about caring for your body through your diet *before* disease occurs? Nutrients are meant to restore and optimize normal function, not alter it. This is not to say we need to ingest a multitude of supplements to achieve optimal micronutrient status. The point here is to recognize optimal micronutrients aren't going to be found in prepackaged "fortified" foods. Rather, the consumption of a multitude and variety of plant-based foods is the key. It's the immunity food fix!

START WITH CELLS

The human body is complex: Cells collected together create your tissue. Several tissues together make up your organs. Organs working together create organ systems, and all your organ systems collectively result in the organism that is you. Nourishing your body at the cellular level speaks to how your body will respond in health or disease.

Your body needs nutrients for communication between the cells of different organ systems. Each part of this process has a specific structure that dictates the function. And every disease likely is a cellular dysfunction, regardless of the symptoms. Simply put, every diagnosable condition has something going on with the cells. If our cells are receiving the nutrients they need, then they should all be healthy—which translates to healthy tissue, organs, organ system, and thus a healthy YOU!

Our cells also require optimal nutrients to survive and thrive. Nutrients keep the cells healthy and operating. The majority of this energy is made by the mitochondria, our source of energy that allows every cell in our body do what that it is supposed to do. Both macro- and micronutrients are important for energy production.

The importance of mitochondria goes beyond energy production, however. Mitochondria is known as the powerhouse of the cell and is involved in both differentiation and activation of our immune cells. When immune cells are activated, they require a lot of energy to carry out their processes. Increasing mitochondrial function is the key mechanism for generating energy for T regulatory cells.

Mitochondria also impact immune cells through their ability to generate reactive oxygen species (ROS). ROS are a bad thing when we think about the damaging effects they have on our DNA and the need to balance that with antioxidant-rich foods. But it's a little more complex than that. Some ROS are always found within the body and are used to maintain homeostatic balance in the body.

The problem is when we have ROS that out-number antioxidants. When this happens, intracellular oxidation causes damage to cell membranes, DNA, and RNA. The activation of the inflammatory cascade is a double-edged sword: the inflammation response leads to the production of reactive oxygen species, which are used to destroy invading pathogens (the bad guys) but can also damage healthy tissue when in a high inflammatory state.

ROS are generated in the mitochondria as a by-product of the conversion of calories and oxygen into the body's usable energy source. What does that mean? It tells us the most important factor in balancing ROS is *diet*. Dietary antioxidants can protect mitochondrial damage. We support our mitochondria with micronutrients and macronutrients, and create the balance with antioxidants from our diet. It goes back to everything being about *balance*.

Keep in mind that we are all individuals, and we all require variable amounts of vitamins and nutrients depending on our genetic makeup. The current conventional nutritional recommendations do not take this into account. And new evidence identifies suboptimal nutrient status as linked to epidemic disease such as osteoporosis, cancer, cardiovascular disease, and autoimmune disorders.

Ideally, we want to obtain our micronutrient content from the foods we eat. Getting to those optimal levels can be a struggle. Conventional farming, nutrient soil depletion, and pesticide use have changed the nutrient content of our food. The term "hidden hunger" has been used to describe nutritional deficiencies that occur when people consume adequate calories but inadequate micronutrients.

hidden hunger

Hidden hunger is more widespread than you might think. Large nationally representative surveys indicate that the intake of certain nutrients in the United States falls below the Institute of Medicine's Estimated Average Requirement (EAR).

Data from 2003 through 2006 showed that (excluding supplements) the total usual intake from food sources fell significantly short:

» Vitamin A: 45 percent

» Vitamin C: 37 percent

» Vitamin D: 93 percent

» Vitamin E: 91 percent

» Calcium: 49 percent

» Magnesium: 55 percent

Remember: Most nutrients act in all tissues. And all tissues need all nutrients. Inadequate intake may adversely affect every body system, but with more pronounced effects in some than others.

WHY IS THIS IMPORTANT? MACRONUTRIENTS AND YOUR IMMUNE SYSTEM

When we think about designing our dietary lifestyle there needs to be a balance between micronutrients, macronutrients, and phytochemicals. This balance helps mitigate the development of disease. In *Immunity Food Fix*, we discussed different types of carbohydrates, the balance of fats, and the importance of protein. These macronutrients are essential to the human body and provide us with the energy and nutrients we need to function. They are required by the body for physiological processes and energy production.

When we think about our "macros" (protein, fat, and carbohydrates), we associate them with diets, weight loss, and muscle building. But macros are essential for so much more. Much like micronutrients, they play a critical role in the function of our immune system. Let's take a look at each macronutrient and break down these details.

PROTEIN

Protein gets a lot of focus, especially in the diet industry, for its role in weight loss and building muscle. Protein is important, but so are fats and carbohydrates. Nutritious nuts and supporting seeds are high in natural plant protein that supports our health.

Proteins are made up of amino acids, and the majority of our body and the messengers within our body are made up of amino acids. This includes, RNA, DNA, hormones, neurotransmitters, and most of our muscles. Protein is an important building block for every cell in our body, and they are made up of essential and nonessential amino acids.

There are nine essential amino acids that we must get from foods. Seek out foods containing all the essential amino acids, or combine your foods to make sure you get what you need. This balance supports all the metabolic reactions in our body, from our immune response to cellular repair and detoxification.

A deficiency in dietary protein impairs your immune function, making you more prone to disease. This is especially a problem in most developing countries where protein deficiency has an impact on the immune response and thus disease development.

The various amino acids impact the body's immune response either directly or indirectly. We refer to antibodies and cytokines as proteins as well, and therefore they require sufficient amino acids in order to be made. These are critical for various metabolic pathways as well as to fight infection.

When you consume protein, your digestive system breaks it down into smaller amino acids. These amino acids are used by the different systems in the body, and are broken down further by enzymes and cofactors to allow them to perform different functions.

Amino acids have a few key roles in immune system regulation and function. Amino acids are necessary to activate natural killer cells. Natural killer (NK) cells are an important part of the innate or nonspecific immune system, where they work to contain viral infections before the adaptive immune system kicks in. They are also needed to activate macrophages, B cells, and T cells in response to a foreign invader. Amino acids are needed to activate the release of cytokines. Amino

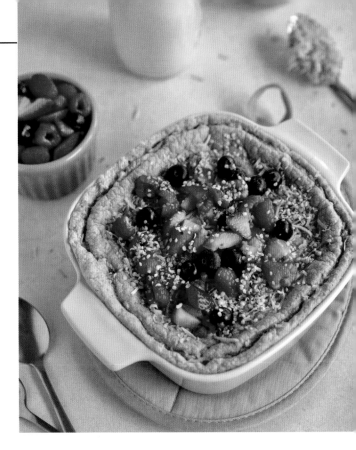

Baked Oatmeal with
Mixed Berries, page 110

acids from protein are also important to balance antioxidant and oxidative stress—the redox state. This helps reduce chronic inflammation and mitigate the development of disease.

Remember, our body cannot make all these amino acids. We need to get essential amino acids from our diet. Additionally, our body does not store protein, so continuous and consistent consumption is important. You can refer to the *Immunity Food Fix* to gain a better understanding of essential versus nonessential profiles of amino acids, especially in plants.

→ GREAT FOOD SOURCES: **Quinoa, lentils, chickpeas, nuts, seeds, tofu**

→ START HERE: **You will love the protein-packed Creamy Chicken and Rice Soup with Basil and Lemon (page 156). Believe it or not, you are getting 30 grams of protein in a bowl of soup!**

FATS

Unfortunately, we have been battling the question of whether fat is good for us for about thirty years. This all started in the 1990s, when the National Institutes of Health associated fat intake with the development of heart disease. What was missing in this notion was the fact that not all fats are created equal. This led to the low-fat diet movement, and the push to consume highly inflammatory fats such as canola oil as an alternative.

As the food industry developed, the American lifestyle shifted and a need for convenient food rose. This led to an increase in exposure to inflammatory and processed fatty acids and less anti-inflammatory fats (omega-3s). We now understand the importance of consuming healthy fats rich in omega-3s to reduce inflammation.

Saturated fats are really the main fat we want to avoid. Omega-6 fatty acids are considered inflammatory, but it is more the *balance* between omega-3 and omega-6 that is important, as we do need some omega-6 fatty acids in the body. Research has found that saturated fatty acids promote lipopolysaccharide (LPS) to translocate from the gut and leak into the bloodstream, stimulating an innate immune response. LPS is toxic to humans.

Studies have shown that continuous high-fat diets elevate levels of these toxins in the blood, which disrupts the gut bacteria and leads to elevated levels of inflammatory cytokines. By consuming fat that is high in MUFAs and PUFAs as opposed to saturated fatty acids, we can mitigate the inflammatory effect of LPS and trigger the innate immune system to respond.

So why are MUFAs and PUFAs that we find in nuts, seeds, and oils so important? Our unsaturated fatty acids (PUFAs and MUFAs) are broken down into two groups, omega-6 (linolenic acid) and omega-3 (alpha-linoleic acid) fatty acids. These unsaturated fatty acids are known to alter immune cell function because they play a direct role in cell composition, and they enhance immune function through various processes.

Dietary PUFAs play an important role in our innate and adaptive immune responses. Much of the research is focused on omega-3 fatty acids (ALA) and EPA and DHA. These fatty acids inhibit the activation of immune cells in the innate and adaptive immune systems. Omega-3 fatty acids have a positive effect on certain immune cells and an impact on T regulatory cells.

→ **GREAT FOOD SOURCES: Mustard seeds, chia seeds, bok choy, salmon**

→ **START HERE: Check out the Golden Coconut Tofu Bowls with Bok Choy and Broccoli (page 148) or the Roasted Cabbage with Chicken and Mustard Seed Sauce (page 163) as a great source of omega-3 fatty acids.**

CARBOHYDRATES

Carbohydrates serve multiple purposes. They are critical for our gut health and mitigating dysbiosis. Carbohydrates are compounds that contain a carbon, a hydrogen, and an oxygen. They are found in sugars, starches, and cellulose. Carbohydrates are classified as:

» Sugars and starches

» Simple and complex

» Minimally processed versus highly processed

Carbohydrates have gotten a bad reputation, but we need the right carbohydrates. Processed carbohydrates have a negative impact on our immune system and our gut health. They cause excess inflammation in the body, alter the gut microbiome, and decrease short-chain fatty acid production. Good starchy carbohydrates—think fruits and vegetables—are loaded with fiber, which is essential to support our gut bacteria and in turn supports our immune system.

Dietary fiber is important for the production of short-chain fatty acids (SCFAs). SCFAs are the essential fuel for the epithelial cells that line our intestines. Recent literature has found that butyrate, a particular SCFA, has important functions in our intestinal tract and immunomodulatory functions.

There are three well-studied SCFAs: acetate, propionate, and butyrate. Their mechanism is to suppress the growth of pathogenic bacteria by lowering intestinal pH, and they help regulate metabolism and the immune system. SCFAs play a role in our immune response through their ability to control the growth of bad bacteria while helping our good bacteria flourish.

» Acetic acid serves as an energy substrate for the liver.

» Propionic acid participates in gluconeogenesis.

» Butyric acid promotes the induction of regulatory T cells in the large intestine.

Butyrate in particular has been found to reduce leaky gut (permeability) via its ability to regulate occludin and zonulin. These proteins help regulate the tight junction of the cells lining the GI tract to prevent foreign invaders from entering and hold together those tight junctions. Another important role they play is modulating mucus thickness in the gut mucosa. Increasing mucus production in the gut helps create that barrier in the gut wall to limit the invasion of external pathogens (bad guys). When you have low mucus production in the gut, you get an imbalance in your good and bad bacteria and, ultimately, leaky gut.

Short-chain fatty acids play a critical role in reducing inflammation through T regulatory cells. Many studies have shown that T regulatory cells are depending on the gut microbiota for proper development and function. It's been found that SCFAs are key to promote differentiation of naïve T cells into T regulatory calls in the intestine. When these SCFAs interact with naïve T cells they lead to the development of T regulatory cells. Some early research in animals has found that SCFAs may play a role in mitigating cells producing autoantibodies and thereby reduce the development of autoimmune diseases.

Lastly, SCFAs play a critical role in glucose regulation and gut hormones. This is important as we consider bringing all the pieces together. Fiber-rich diets high in SCFAs lead to an increase in circulating gut hormones such as GLP-1 and PYY. GLP-1 has a unique mechanism responsible for releasing insulin, inhibiting glucagon, and delaying gastric emptying after a meal is ingested. PYY is a gut peptide released in response to food more related to fat and protein. It has been shown to reduce appetite by slowing gastric emptying. This increases efficiency of digestion and nutrient absorption after a meal.

→ GREAT FOOD SOURCES: Chickpeas provide the gut with butyrate, a key SCFA. Potatoes are an excellent source of resistant starch that forms SCFAs and feeds our gut.

→ START HERE: Check out the Lemony Shrimp Chickpea Pasta with Spinach and Walnuts (page 160) to feed your microbiome. Craving potatoes? Try the Spiced Lentils with Tomatoes and Red Potatoes (page 144)!

WHY IS THIS IMPORTANT? MICRONUTRIENTS AND YOUR IMMUNE SYSTEM

When we think about immunity, most of us immediately think, "Take some vitamin C." And vitamin C does play a role, but there is a much longer list of micronutrients that are essential to immunity. In fact, the three mechanisms within our immune system—mucosal, innate, and adaptive—require various micronutrients to carry out every stage of the immune response.

MUCOSAL IMMUNE SYSTEM

Starting with our first line of defense, we know that iron is important for differentiation of growth of epithelial tissue. We also know that vitamin A and

THE BREAKDOWN OF MICRONUTRIENTS
in the Various Stages of Immune Response

Mucosal	Innate	Adaptive
Vitamin A	Vitamin A	Vitamin A
Vitamin D	Vitamin D	Vitamin D
Vitamin C	Vitamin C	Vitamin C
Vitamin E	Vitamin E	Vitamin E
Vitamin B_6	Vitamin B_6	Vitamin B_6
Vitamin B_{12}	Vitamin B_{12}	Vitamin B_{12}
Folate	Folate (B_9)	Folate (B_9)
Iron	Zinc	Zinc
Zinc	Iron	Iron
	Copper	Copper
	Selenium	Selenium
	Magnesium	Magnesium

zinc are critical in the structural and functional integrity of the skin and mucosal cells. (Vitamin A for IgA—the key antibody produced by our mucosal immune system.)

The balance between the good and bad bacteria in our gut is affected by vitamin D, A, B_6, B_{12}, and folate. These vitamins increase the concentrations of Bifidobacterium, the key microbe involved in increasing our T regulatory cells.

Vitamin D also plays a unique role in stimulating tight junction protein expression in the gut. Those tight junctions need to be controlled to maintain the intestinal barrier, which is porous enough to absorb necessary nutrients but tight enough to stop antigens from flowing into the bloodstream and generating an immune response.

Collagen production supports and strengthens our gut lining. It also helps increase SCFA production, which supplies up to 70 percent of the energy used by colonic epithelial cells and promotes intestinal mucosal cell regeneration.

Vitamin C is necessary for the promotion of collagen synthesis in the epithelial gut lining, which is critical to allow for nutrient absorption and phytochemicals. So, it all goes hand in hand. Vitamins C and E are also important antioxidants, which protect the cell membranes from damage by free radicals.

INNATE IMMUNE SYSTEM

Here are a few examples of this incredible response team:

» Interferon defends the body by preventing viral replication. Selenium is a key nutrient that helps increase interferon production; vitamin C, zinc, and iron also play important roles.

» Natural killer (NK) cells work to contain viral infections. Vitamin A regulates the expression and the amount of NK cells, and vitamins B_6, B_{12}, C, E, folate, and zinc make them stronger (enhancing their killing potential).

» Macrophages are a type of white blood cell that surrounds and kills microorganisms. They also remove dead cells and stimulate the action of other immune system cells. Macrophages contain a significant amount of iron.

ADAPTIVE IMMUNITY

When the innate immune response cannot fight off a pathogen, it asks for help. The adaptive (specific) immune system develops over time, and we can think of it as the "special forces." Turning on the adaptive immune system activates our T cells and B cells. They figure out what the pathogen is and give a more directed approach to kill it off. It's a much slower process, but the system also has a good memory. This keeps us from getting reinfected with the same pathogen over and over again.

The two T helper cells I want you to remember are TH1 and TH2. TH1 cells are key in the immune

anemia of inflammation

Systemic immune activation leads to changes of iron trafficking within the body, which results in two things:

» Iron retention in macrophages

» Reduced dietary iron absorption

How does this occur, exactly? Systemic inflammation results in immune cell activation and the formation of numerous cytokines. These cytokines are potent inducers of hepcidin, an iron-regulating hormone made in the liver, and it controls delivery of iron to the blood.

Hepcidin causes iron retention in macrophages and blocks dietary iron absorption in the intestine. When you have elevated levels due to elevated inflammation, you have more iron retention in the macrophages and less absorbed in the intestines. This leads to efficient iron storage but inefficient iron export.

Macrophages are activated by pro-inflammatory cytokines; their production is regulated by vitamin A. Vitamin D helps create balance here by reducing the expression of pro-inflammatory cytokines and increasing anti-inflammatory cytokines. Just another reason why vitamin D is so important in creating balance in the immune response.

response against bacteria, viruses, and tumor cells. For this reason, it should be no surprise that when TH1 is activated it releases inflammatory cytokines to fight that foreign invader. So remember, TH1 response is associated with inflammation. TH2 cells are activated in response to allergies or parasites.

Which nutrients are most important to support these activation processes within the adaptive immune system? Here's a short list:

» Vitamin A is responsible for the development and differentiation of TH1 and TH2 cells. Gosh, all I've ever heard about vitamin A is its importance in eye health, but at every stage of immunity it's responsible for development and differentiation of key cells.

» Vitamin E works to suppress the TH2 inflammatory response.

---

t cells

These cells have a variety of functions. Think of them as the helpers, the killers, and the regulators.

» **Helper T cells indirectly kill a foreign invader.**

» **Cytotoxic T cells directly kill the foreign invader with no additional help.**

» **T regulatory cells control the process and suppress inappropriate reactions.**

» Vitamin B_6, folate, and zinc work to maintain the TH1 response when it's needed.

» Vitamin D and zinc are critical in promoting the development of T regulatory cells, which help calm the immune system. Increasing T regulatory cells can help "regulate" or balance T helper cells, reducing the release of inflammatory cytokines.

While we want to keep it simple by focusing on TH1 as the inflammatory helper cells, I also want you to be aware of TH17. TH1 and TH17 both produce pro-inflammatory cytokines that are associated with the development of autoimmune disorders.

Antibody development requires amino acids to be synthesized, so to support them they require the B vitamins for their development. While B vitamins are needed for synthesis of antibodies, vitamin C helps increase serum levels. Other nutrients involved in antibody production include copper, selenium, magnesium, and zinc.

It's clear to see that micronutrients in general are necessary for the activation and function of the immune system. When levels are low, we impact our immune system's ability to respond as necessary. Each particular nutrient plays a specific role, yet they all work in harmony to get the job done!

VITAMIN C

Vitamin C plays a critical role in the immune system and at all stages of the immune response. It supports the integrity of the gut wall by promoting collagen synthesis and protects cell membranes from free radical damage. Its antioxidant properties also protect leukocytes and lymphocytes from oxidative stress.

When we have a lack of vitamin C, we get increased oxidative damage, impaired wound healing, and increased incidence of infections such as pneumonia.

→ GREAT FOOD SOURCES: **Citrus fruits, kiwi-fruit, tomatoes, peppers, Brussels sprouts**

→ START HERE: **Citrus Olive Salad with Shrimp • Edamame, and Cilantro Vinaigrette (page 128) • Crispy Miso Brussels Sprouts and Tempeh over Quinoa with Sage and Almond Butter Sauce (page 142) • Passion Fruit Panna Cotta (page 179)**

VITAMIN D

Vitamin D is so critical to immune health, specifically to increasing our T regulatory cells. These cells prevent the body from reacting to nonharmful substances, and they are also responsible for the prevention of an autoimmune response.

Vitamin D also is responsible for increasing tight junction protein expression in the gut wall, which ultimately leads to less leaky gut. Other key attributes are its ability to activate macrophages and reduce cytokine expression, which are typically due to an inflammatory response.

→ GREAT FOOD SOURCES: **Cod liver oil and fatty fish. The best way to get adequate vitamin D is through the sun!**

→ START HERE: **Cantaloupe and Smoked Salmon Caprese with Lemon-Mint Pesto (page 53) • Green Tea Rice Bowls with Miso-Glazed Salmon (page 71) • Moroccan-Spiced Carrot and Parsnip Salad with Lemon-Roasted Cod (page 158)**

VITAMIN A

Vitamin A is so important for our mucosal immune system. We want to maintain a high level of IgA in our mucosal barriers; a low level of IgA translates to a leaky gut. IgA also helps increase T regulatory cells and maintains tolerance across the immune system.

Vitamin A also has been found to improve antibody titer response to vaccines. Basically, it means when you get vaccinated, having adequate vitamin A correlates to a better immune response to the vaccine. Interesting, huh?

→ GREAT FOOD SOURCES: **Liver, fish oil, eggs; also found in carrots, cantaloupe, spinach**

→ START HERE: **Carrot-Ginger Spice Spelt Muffins (page 69) • Butternut Scramble over Mixed Greens (page 103) • Grounding Daily Kichadi (page 109) • Pumpkin Cardamom Oats with Coconut Butter and Orange Zest (page 90)**

VITAMIN E

Vitamin E is an excellent antioxidant. It protects cell membranes from free radical damage and supports the integrity of the epithelial barriers. It impacts and improves overall immune function.

→ GREAT FOOD SOURCES: **Green leafy vegetables, sunflower seeds, almonds**

→ START HERE: **Egg Muffins with Butternut and Sunflower Seed Pesto (page 106) • Blue Fried Rice with Salmon (page 168) • Passion Fruit Panna Cotta (page 179)**

B VITAMINS

Each B vitamin plays a unique role. Vitamin B_6 helps restore and support adaptive immune system. Vitamin B_{12} has a similar role, and it's also critical for gut health. Vitamin B_9 (folate) can help increase innate immunity. It also supports a TH1 response; these cells work against bacteria, viruses, and tumor cells.

→ **GREAT FOOD SOURCES OF B_6: Chickpeas, liver, tuna, bananas**

→ **GREAT FOOD SOURCES OF B_{12}: Liver, bananas, fish**

→ **GREAT FOOD SOURCES OF B_9: Dark leafy vegetable, beans, seeds, seafood**

→ **START HERE: Tuna, Chickpea, and Arugula Salad with Lemon and Tarragon Vinaigrette (page 123) • Chickpea, Edamame, and Salmon Salad with Lemon Basil-Dill Vinaigrette (page 127) • Minty Mango Green Smoothie (page 95)**

ZINC

Zinc deficiency has a direct impact on the number of T cells and the activity of NK (natural killer) cells. This is critical because without zinc your immune cells don't mature and develop the way they are intended to. Zinc is critical for the activation of cells in both the innate and the adaptive immune system. Zinc status has a direct effect on T cell functions and the balance between the different T helper cell subsets. Acute zinc deficiency causes a decrease in innate and adaptive immunity; chronic deficiency increases inflammation.

→ **GREAT FOOD SOURCES: Meat, legumes, shellfish, oysters, hemp seeds, flaxseeds, pumpkin seeds, nuts (especially cashews), eggs, whole grains, dairy products, dark chocolate, potatoes**

→ **START HERE: Papaya and Coconut Yogurt Breakfast Bowls (page 101) • Cabbage Salad Lettuce Wraps with Spicy Chicken (page 130) • Smoky Black Bean and Butternut Tacos with Pumpkin Seeds (page 140)**

IRON

Iron is the most common nutrient deficiency around the world. It's essential that your iron levels are just right; you don't want too much or too little.

Iron deficiency leads to impaired cellular immunity, decreased T helper cells, and lower levels of IL-6, which are needed to fight pathogens in time of need. Remember, the T helper cells work by indirectly killing a foreign invader by either directly releasing cytokines or by telling B cells to prepare the response with antibodies.

→ **GREAT FOOD SOURCES: Spinach, lentils, beans, nuts**

→ **START HERE: Southwestern Quinoa Salad with Yellow Squash and Black Beans (page 73) • Everyday Veggie Egg Bake (page 105) • Chicken Radicchio Salad with Apple, Celery, and Cashews with Apricot Dressing (page 119)**

SELENIUM

Selenium is an essential nutrient involved in many redox reactions, making it critical as an antioxidant. Given its antioxidant function, it protects immune cells from oxidative stress as well. Selenium improves the response in adaptive immunity and improves T helper cell counts, allowing for an enhanced immune response to viruses in deficient individuals.

Selenium content in the diet can vary significantly depending on the amount of selenium present in the soil and taken up by the plants (foods). Less than optimal intake of selenium has been found in various regions in Europe and the Eastern Mediterranean due to the selenium-poor soils.

→ GREAT FOOD SOURCES: **Brazil nuts, oysters, tuna, whole-wheat bread, sunflower seeds, pork, beef, lamb, turkey, mushrooms, rye**

→ START HERE: **Kale Salad with Chicken and Sweet Chlorella Dressing (page 134) • Roasted Cabbage with Chicken and Mustard Seed Sauce (page 163) • Roasted Asparagus Salad with Tempeh, White Beans, and Radish in Lemon Zest Vinaigrette with Brazil Nut Crumble (page 152)**

MAGNESIUM

Magnesium is a common and imperative mineral in the body involved in more than 600 enzymatic reactions. Magnesium deficiency is associated with increased inflammation and recurrent bacterial infections. It plays a role in antigen binding to macrophages, so you can see why low magnesium can lead to increased infections. Magnesium is also a cofactor in antibody synthesis, meaning you need it to make antibodies!

→ GREAT FOOD SOURCES: **Green leafy vegetables (spinach), legumes (black beans, edamame), nuts, seeds (pumpkin, chia)**

→ START HERE: **Tahini Chocolate Chip Cookies (page 183), Sweet Potato Sunchoke Dip (page 66), Sprouted Quinoa Porridge with Raspberries and Hazelnut Butter (page 89)**

COPPER

Copper plays an important role in the immune system, being both anti-inflammatory and antioxidant in nature. Low copper can lead to ineffective immune response to infections and increase viral virulence. Adequate copper allows for the ability to scavenge free radicals as well as antimicrobial properties. It plays a role in the innate immune response to bacterial infections.

→ GREAT FOOD SOURCES: **Shellfish, seeds, nuts, organ meats, whole grains, chocolate**

→ START HERE: **Chickpea, Edamame, and Salmon Salad with Lemon Basil-Dill Vinaigrette (page 127) • Smoky Black Bean and Butternut Tacos with Pumpkin Seeds (page 140) • Chocolate-Almond and Rose Cups (page 176)**

EATING FOR HEALTH

As you can see, macronutrients and micronutrients play a critical role in our immune health. Now you combine that with phytonutrients and you can see the benefits that plant-based foods have on your immune and gut health. The recipes in this book combine these plant-based foods to bring these benefits to life in their various synergies.

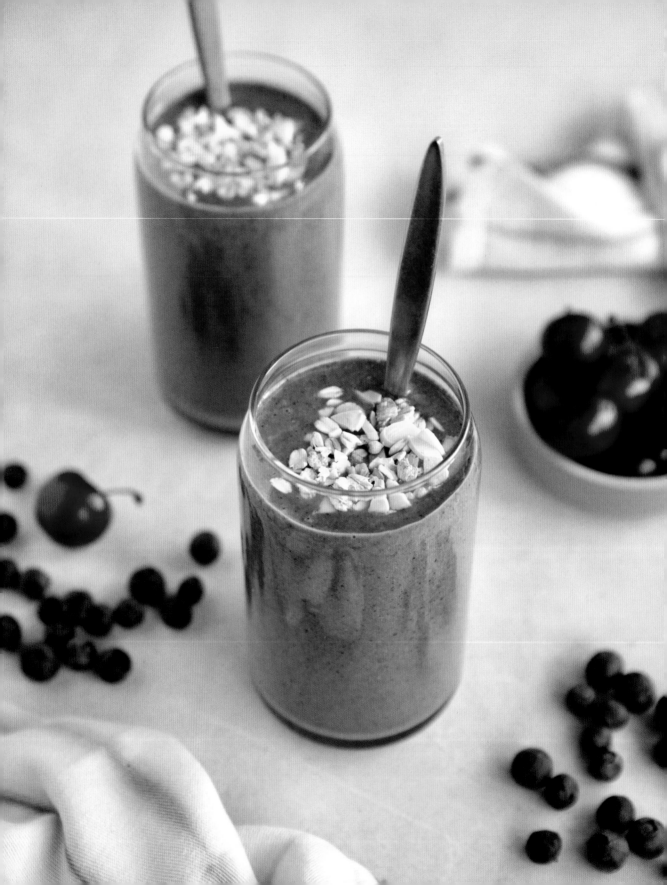

CHAPTER THREE

IMMUNO-METABOLISM & METABOLIC FLEXIBILITY

Immunometabolism describes the changes that occur in various metabolic pathways within our immune cells. These changes alter the function of the cells—in the wrong way! By continuously eating inflammatory foods, we are shifting the way our immune system responds to disease and self-tissue. Our gut microbiota and gut wall play a critical role in determining disease development. In this chapter, we will learn about glucose dysregulation and the impact it has on the development of metabolic and immunologic diseases.

Banana-Blueberry-Cherry
Smoothie, page 97

IMMUNOMETABOLISM

Okay, you've learned about your immune system and how various nutrients and phytochemicals impact immunity. Now let's tie it all together with what you eat. Immunometabolism may be a new term for you, but it really ties in your immune system and your metabolic pathways.

There are two aspects to consider about immunometabolism. One is the effect of inflammation and immune response on the overall systemic metabolism. The other is the nitty-gritty of the effects of metabolism on inflammation within immune cells.

Now let's expand to talk about immunometabolism. When your immune system is triggered, your body requires energy to fight that trigger. Enter your metabolism. If your metabolic health is lacking, you may not be able to support that immune function. And vice versa.

A focus on a healthy lifestyle, eating enough of the right foods, and getting enough exercise can boost your metabolic health. This, in turn, improves your immune health. In the case of autoimmune disease, shifting your immune response through metabolic changes can help support your immune response for the better.

YOUR METABOLISM

Your metabolism gives you the energy you need to function. That energy comes from the foods you eat and drink. When your body converts food, it creates the energy you burn.

Think about this in terms of three different processes:

1 BASAL METABOLISM: 60–80 percent of calories burned

2 THERMIC EFFECT OF FOOD: 10 percent of calories burned

3 PHYSICAL ACTIVITY: 10–30 percent of calories burned

Your basal metabolism is used for your functions, and it burns the majority of your calories in a day. We refer to this as your basal metabolic rate, the energy you burn while at rest. Thermic effect of food is the amount of energy your body needs to break down the food you eat. Physical activity is the energy burned when you exercise.

IMMUNOMETABOLISM AND CHRONIC INFLAMMATION

Let's start with obesity as a cause for chronic inflammation, and inflammation as the root of disease. We know that plants contain bioactive compounds that reduce chronic inflammation and produce an antioxidant effect. They have proven to support immune function and prevent disease development. But the majority of the population is consuming an inflammatory, which leads to glucose dysregulation and obesity. And we now know that chronic inflammation, especially that in adipose (fat) tissue and the liver, plays a significant role in insulin resistance and glucose intolerance.

Metabolism-induced inflammation associated with obesity is termed *metainflammation*. The Western diet is a known risk factor. It is high in sugar, trans fats, and saturated fats, but low in complex carbohydrates, fiber, micronutrients, and other bioactive molecules (such as polyphenols and omega-3 polyunsaturated fatty acids). These are all things we now know we need to avoid in order to improve our metabolic health.

WHAT IS METABOLIC HEALTH?

We hear this term a lot, especially during the pandemic, when someone's immune response wasn't as strong due to poor metabolic health, as seen in individuals with high blood pressure and diabetes. Simply put, metabolic health means having ideal blood sugar levels, cholesterol levels, blood pressure, and waist circumference. This is tied to an overall healthy weight, endurance when you exercise, and balanced mood and energy.

Poor metabolic health has significant implications for your immune system and overall health. Several studies demonstrate that chronic inflammation from adipose tissue can cause decreased insulin sensitivity and impair insulin secretion. Obesity is significantly related to chronic inflammation: the greater the BMI of an individual, the greater the level of inflammation. This indicates that the incidence of chronic inflammation has increased in direct proportion to the incidence of obesity.

Obesity leads to chronic inflammation in our metabolic tissues, including the liver, adipose tissue, and muscle. It also causes dysbiosis in the gut, the largest component of our mucosal immune system. This chronic inflammatory response in our metabolic tissues results in the release of inflammatory cytokines and results in downstream effects, such as metabolic dysfunction and insulin resistance. This is a problem because then we have higher circulating glucose in the blood and the body trying to produce more insulin to get it out.

Inflammation associated with obesity also plays a role in how our T cells function and change. For example, fatty acid synthesis is essential for TH17 cell differentiation, and we see accumulation in high-fat diets and a reduction in T regulatory cells as a result. This leads to the production of inflammatory cytokine IL-17, which is associated with the development of autoimmunity. The opposite occurs in an anti-inflammatory state, where we see increases in T regulatory cells over TH17 cell development.

Obesity induces a chronic low-grade inflammatory response as a result of diets that contain excess intake of calories, salt, fat, and sugar. This response is associated with higher CRP levels, elevated cytokines. Cytokines released from fat cells are referred to adipokines and are referred to as peptide hormones. Elevations in these hormones leads to insulin resistance and metabolic dysfunction. Interestingly, studies have found that low-grade systemic inflammation measured by elevated CRP levels was found to predict hemoglobin A1C levels, a measure of blood glucose and insulin resistance.

Keep in mind that chronic low-grade inflammation stemming from the adipose tissue leading to insulin resistance is just one part of the equation. The adipose tissue inflammation also influences changes in immune cells leading to an increase and alterations in adipokines and cytokines, which ultimately impacts skeletal muscle and liver insulin resistance. This is a problem because then we have higher circulating glucose in the blood and the body trying to produce more insulin to get it out.

LET'S CONNECT THE DOTS

In chapter 1 we talked about nonalcoholic fatty liver disease (NAFLD). NAFLD is associated with an increase in leaky gut, and this is related to the increased prevalence of gut dysbiosis and small intestinal bacterial overgrowth. The gut dysbiosis and translocation of bacteria across the

ADIPOKINES *(Fat Hormones)*

Leptin	Adiponectin
• Fat cell–derived hormone • Speaks to the hypothalamus to enhance metabolism and reduce appetite • Said to increase sympathetic activity and increase energy expenditure	• Fat cell–derived hormone • Known to be insulin sensitizing and anti-inflammatory • Negatively correlated with BMI • Increased fat cells equate to less adiponectin • Associated with longevity, decreased risk for cardiovascular disease, and decreased risk for diabetes mellitus DM and insulin resistance • Decreases gluconeogenesis • Increases mitochondrial biogenesis • Associated with more beta oxidation (mitochondria to make adenosine triphosphate [ATP])

epithelial barrier increases liver dysfunction, leads to NAFLD, and in turn worsens leaky gut. It's a vicious cycle that keeps going around!

Obesity—on its own—is associated with increased liver inflammation. This inflammation is characterized by the release of macrophages. This smaller family of cytokines referred to as chemokines recruit immune cells into the liver and differentiate into pro-inflammatory macrophages, which leads to insulin resistance.

Now that you understand the role of obesity on NAFLD and metabolic dysfunction, how does the skeletal muscle play a role? Skeletal muscle is responsible for the uptake of 80 percent of glucose from the blood and thus for regulating glucose. An increase in macrophages and systemic inflammation impacts insulin sensitivity and the ability to regulate glucose homeostasis, impacting muscle insulin resistance.

Obesity can also impact the release of various gut hormones, and this, in turn, impacts our immune system. These hormones are both inflammatory and anti-inflammatory. Remember, we said that the cytokines released from fat tissue are referred to as adipokines. These adipokines are further referred to as hormones. The fat tissue controls immune function through the secretion of these hormones (adipokines). The two adipokines we are referring to are leptin, which is pro-inflammatory, and adiponectin, which is anti-inflammatory. Adiponectin is inversely correlated to excess belly fat. The bigger the belly, the lower the adiponectin and the higher the leptin (inflammatory). This is why waist circumference is an important measure of metabolic health.

Adiponectin and leptin play an important role in energy and metabolic homeostasis, and they can be influenced by underlying inflammation. Leptin is one of the most important hormones secreted by fat (adipose tissue). Leptin provides crucial information on the link between metabolic state and immune system function. Leptin was initially thought of as the anti-obesity hormone, but more recent research has shown that it influences the balance between the immune system.

HOW DOES THIS WORK?

If you are overweight, you get a high amount of leptin secreted by adipocytes because of inflammatory conditions. What this means is you get more T cells activated and releasing pro-inflammatory cytokines. It also reduces the number of T regulatory cells, which we know are important to balance the immune system. This imbalance can lead to poor metabolic function, an increased incidence of autoimmune disorders, and chronic inflammation.

Several studies in humans reveal that leptin levels are associated with autoimmune disorders, infections, and endocrine/metabolic diseases. This suggests a central role of leptin in immune balance and in the development of several inflammatory disorders.

Too much leptin in the blood also can lead to leptin resistance. This impairs the body's satiety functions, so your body doesn't know when you are full and can't turn off that hunger hormone. Elevated circulating leptin levels in obesity appear to contribute to the low-grade inflammatory background, meaning that obese individuals may be more susceptible to increased risk of developing cardiovascular diseases, diabetes, or degenerative diseases, including autoimmunity and cancer.

Leptin sits at the interface between metabolism and immunity, modulating inflammation and also immune and autoimmune reactivity. When leptin is high, its anti-inflammatory counterpart, adiponectin, is low. Adiponectin is typically low in overweight individuals. This is a problem because adiponectin is known to be insulin sensitizing, anti-inflammatory, and associated with longevity.

OBESITY AND AUTOIMMUNE DISEASE

Adipose tissue creates a low-grade inflammatory response. Obesity is detrimental to our metabolic health, and it can cause an inflammatory immune response in the body. Research has found that overeating can cause stress and damage to the mitochondria, which is caused by fatty acid buildup in cells. That long-term metainflammation puts prolonged stress on the mitochondria. Overnutrition and overeating are part of the problem. Overnutrition and chronic inflammation put us at risk for disease development. But undernutrition is a concern as well because it is linked to immunosuppression.

HOW CAN WE FIX THIS?

So how do we create a balance? Eating an anti-inflammatory diet and reducing inflammation overall is critical. Remember, the immunity food fix is to consume a variety of plants in a multitude of colors to reduce chronic inflammation with which so many of us live. It's that simple!

We want to maintain our health daily to prevent disease, and we can use food to help fight disease should it arise. Plants contain bioactive compounds that reduce chronic inflammation in the body and produce an antioxidant effect. Plants have a proven ability to support our immune

Anti-Inflammatory Effects of Exercise across Organs

BRAIN

The hypothalamic-pituitary-adrenal axis is activated and induces the adrenal cortex and the medulla to produce cortisol and adrenaline, respectively. These two hormones, in turn, suppress the release of the pro-inflammatory tumor necrosis factor (TNF).

SKELETAL MUSCLE

Contracting muscles are responsible for a complex cascade of processes, which ultimately is anti-inflammatory: increases in IL-6 determine a downregulation of TNF as well as an upregulation of IL-10.

LIVER

Expression of follistatin, another member of TNF superfamily, is markedly increased in the liver following exercise to inhibit myostatin action. This helps improve muscle mass and strength.

ADIPOSE TISSUE

In adipose tissue, a switch from M1 to M2 macrophage phenotype may inhibit the release of the pro-inflammatory cytokines IL-6 and TNF and increase the production of anti-inflammatory cytokines, such as IL-10 and adiponectin. IL-10 may be upregulated by the increased circulating numbers of T regulatory cells.

SPLEEN

Exercise can also lower the expression and activation of toll-like receptor 4 (TLR4), thereby reducing adipose tissue infiltration and other pro-inflammatory cytokines.

---

system function and prevent disease development. The direct effect plants have on our gut health and the immune system translates into a direct effect on disease prevention and overall positive immune health.

Functional foods are foods that have a potentially positive effect on health beyond basic nutrition, promoting optimal health and reducing the risk of disease. With the abundance of research out there it is clear that our diet is the key source of energy, fueling our bodies and our metabolic pathways. Phytonutrients, micronutrients, and macronutrients all play a critical role in shaping our immune response and our gut health, as these food antigens come into contact with the gut bacteria as their first point of contact within the body.

WHAT ABOUT INTERMITTENT FASTING?

In addition to the food we eat, there are other mechanisms to create that balance between immunity and metabolism. Intermittent fasting has gained a lot of popularity over the last few years. There are different versions, but the most popular is a 16:8 fast, where your eating window is 8 hours and your fasting window is 16 hours.

Fasting has been shown to raise adiponectin levels and lower leptin. This is critical because we know it impacts inflammation, insulin sensitivity, and glucose regulation. In addition, this has a role in autoimmunity: Elevated levels of leptin inhibit T regulatory cells, which we know are essential for immune tolerance. It is critical for our body to have the ability to prevent a harmful immune response to a detected foreign substance. This is also known as immune tolerance. Our immune system can suppress the immune response and regulate it, to stop processes that could be damaging to you.

HOW CAN EXERCISE HELP?

Exercise is another way to improve your body's immune response and improve metabolism. Regular exercise reduces fat mass and adipose tissue inflammation, which is known to contribute to systemic inflammation. Exercise also increases muscle production of IL-6, which is known to reduce TNF-alpha (inflammatory) and increase anti-inflammatory cytokines. Exercise can down-regulate toll-like receptors, which activates pro-inflammatory cascades.

Exercise training has beneficial effects across a broad spectrum of organ systems, and its anti-inflammatory actions are complicated by the intricate interplay among organs and cytokines.

Exercise suppresses inflammatory cytokine and increases anti-inflammatory cytokines across several organs. (See page 38).

GLUCOSE DYSREGULATION

Let's talk about sugar. I'm not saying all sugar is bad. However, processed sugars that spike glucose in our blood are problematic. When blood sugar is high, the body produces more free radicals that trigger the immune system, damage cells, and cause inflammation in the blood vessels. Also, insulin is released in response to elevated sugar levels to get the sugar out of the blood. An increase in insulin response and release equals increased inflammation.

Have you ever taken the time to track how much added sugar you consume? Read those labels, do the math, and reflect on how that's impacting your immune response. The amount of sugar consumption recommended by the World Health Organization (WHO) Office of Disease Prevention is no more than 10 percent of your daily calories from added sugar, or a limit of 6 teaspoons (roughly 25 grams) of sugar.

It is important to make a distinction between different types of sugars. One way to consider the impact of sugars in our food is by their glycemic index. This is a measure of how much food sugars affect your blood glucose levels. Foods with a high glycemic index lead to spikes in blood glucose immediately after a meal.

Our body processes sugar differently, and the culprit here is really those hidden and refined sugars we find in processed foods and drinks. These sugars have the fiber and phytonutrients removed from them. These are found in crackers, cakes, cookies, cereals, and pretty much just about anything found in a package on your grocery store shelf.

Refined sugars don't have any benefits; they are simply just BAD! As we've evolved our diet, we have reduced the amount of complex carbohydrates and fiber but increased simple sugars. This increase in simple sugars has led to an alteration in our gut microbiota, evolving it in a negative way. This has led to declines in Bifidobacterium in the gut, which is necessary to increase T regulatory cells.

Excess sugar intake has a negative impact on our intestinal mucous barrier. One study showed high sugar consumption can lead to a thinning of the mucous layer that protects the lining of the large intestine and leads to dysbiosis in the gut. Bacteria known to produce mucous membrane–degrading enzymes, such as muciniphila and *Bacteroides fragilis*, were found in HIGH numbers. Other types of bugs considered good bacteria and commonly found in the gut, such as Lactobacillus, became significantly less abundant. What's even more shocking is that the alteration in the gut bacteria and lining occurred within seven days of the high sugar consumption.

THE METABOLIC EFFECTS OF CONSUMING REFINED SUGARS

It's important to remember that eating too much of any type of sugar will ultimately spike your blood glucose level. Your body responds by releasing insulin to pull the sugar from the blood. When we consume excess amounts of sugar, or we continuously operate in a state of elevated blood glucose, our body can't keep up. The cells responsible for releasing insulin become more resistant than sensitive

what does sugar do to your body?

How does this relate to your immune health? Sugar suppresses your immune system, period. In a 2021 study, elevated fructose intake was shown to cause the immune system to release more inflammatory cytokines. We know that the increase in these inflammatory cytokines can lead to inflammation in the body, further leading to damaged cells, tissues, and eventually organs.

Eating high-sugar foods has been found to suppress the immune system for hours after eating depending on how much was consumed. A nutrition study showed that it takes about 75 grams of sugar to weaken the immune system, and it lowers the response for about 5 hours after consumption.

Eating refined sugars causes your blood sugar to rise quickly and activate an enzyme called protein kinase C. This enzyme leads to dysfunction in neutrophils, a type of white blood cell that travels to the source of an infection and then destroys the invading microorganism.

Sugars from whole fruit include the fiber and various phytonutrients. These work with your immune system, not against it.

and therefore your blood sugar level continues to rise. This state of insulin resistance is inflammatory and impacts your immune response. This leads to glucose dysregulation, which is exactly what it says: your body's inability to regulate glucose.

High levels of blood sugar can lead to the production of free radicals, which we know damage our cells and DNA. High blood sugar also can lead to oxidation of free fatty acids, which leads to inflammation. It increases blood vessel constriction, which can lead to blood clots. High glucose can also impact bad cholesterol, LDL, by oxidizing it and increasing plaque buildup.

Excess fat, and the hormones released from fat, lead to increased inflammation and a negative immune response. Excess sugar leads to weight gain, which leads to excess fat—and round and round we go!

ACHIEVING METABOLIC FLEXIBILITY

Metabolic flexibility is the ability to adapt to change in metabolic demand. It is the ability to change our fuel source, either carbs or fats, in different states, such as when fasting, when exercising, while sedentary, or after a meal. If you are metabolically flexible, when you eat, insulin levels rise in response to glucose (carbohydrates). Then your levels decline after you eat. When insulin is low, your body uses fat for energy as opposed to carbs. In addition, when you exercise, your body has the ability to switch to fat stores for energy, allowing you to more easily burn fat.

If you are metabolically inflexible, I want you to remember the concept of insulin resistance. Studies have found that individuals with a higher carb-to-fat burning ratio, meaning they burn carbs regardless of activity, and can't ever tap into those fat stores.

In short, if you eat poorly or rely on the standard American diet, there is a greater likelihood of metabolic inflexibility, along with insulin resistance, increased inflammation, poor gut health, the inability to respond to infection because of a poor immune system, and an inability to achieve optimal health overall.

CARING FOR YOUR METABOLISM

Immunity is our body's ability to fight off a foreign invader, but we need to pay attention to the processes that regulate our immune system. You want them activated when necessary and disarmed when needed, ready for the next attack. It's clear that the systems within our body don't work in silos. They depend on each other to communicate various messages for optimal health. The crosstalk between our immune system and our metabolism is critical for sustaining health, warding off disease, fighting infection, and living our best life.

Our diet, lifestyle, and environment play a key role in our metabolic and immune health. As we focus on how they interact, it allows us to address causes of disease. We can limit the consumption of refined, processed inflammatory foods; this improves insulin sensitivity, gut hormones and bacteria, and metabolic flexibility. The ultimate goal to is to eat whole foods and, as you'll see, the recipes in this book are rich in phytonutrients, macronutrients, and micronutrients. They're delicious and they'll help your body become (and stay!) metabolically healthy.

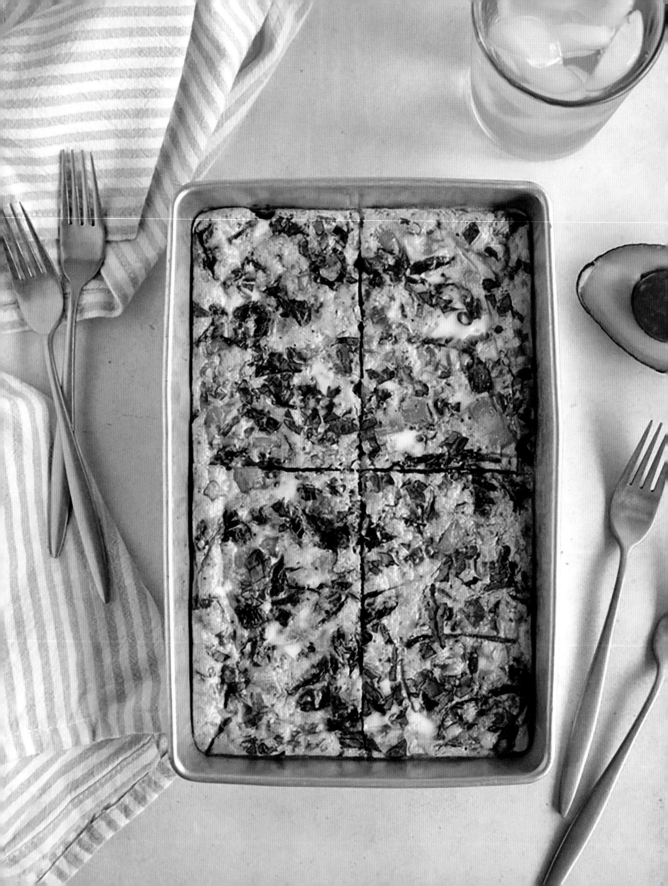

CHAPTER FOUR

EAT TO HEAL & PREVENT DISEASE

Your immune system is so important. In this chapter, we'll look at how food can give your body the nutrients it needs to keep your metabolic processes on track, while also slowing and preventing disease. Pretty amazing, isn't it? Let's pull it all together and learn how to eat to heal!

Everyday Veggie Egg Bake,
page 105

YOU ARE WHAT YOU EAT!

What you eat matters. Our metabolic processes and immunity are all connected, and systemic, chronic, low-grade inflammation is a common denominator in most chronic diseases. It is estimated that one-third of all cancer deaths in the United States could be prevented through dietary modification. According to the World Health Organization, these chronic diseases are responsible for 70 percent of all deaths globally and $47 trillion lost in GDP worldwide. It is recommended by Dietary Guidelines that Americans consume at least nine servings of fruits and vegetables daily. The reality is, the average American consumes 3.6 servings. Let's change that!

PHYTONUTRIENTS, MACRONUTRIENTS, AND MICRONUTRIENTS, OH MY!

PHYTONUTRIENTS

There are still thousands of phytonutrients we haven't identified in plants, whereas we have identified more than 5,000 individual dietary phytochemicals in plant-based foods. While these phytonutrients are so easily accessible, the average person doesn't consume nearly enough to benefit from their properties. Instead of plant-based foods, many of us rely on processed foods that don't help our bodies do what they need to do. And we can't solve this by taking supplements and vitamins to give our bodies the necessary nutrients. We need to consume a variety of whole foods daily and consume them *together*.

That is the beauty of this book and these recipes. I have combined a variety of functional foods, herbs, oils, seeds, and nuts to bring forth that synergy of all these plants working together to gain the overall benefits. Through the various plant-based foods in each recipe, there will be an abundance of phytonutrients made available to the body.

The most important phytonutrients found in plant-based foods are phenolics, alkaloids, nitrogen-containing compounds, organosulfur compounds, phytosterols, and carotenoids. These phytochemicals produce a strong antioxidant and anti-inflammatory effect in the body. But as you'll see in these recipes, we combine a variety of plant-based foods to boost these benefits through the synergy of phytochemicals. This is the greatest benefit of these recipes. You need a balanced diet of a variety of plant-based foods for optimal nutrition, health, and well-being. None of these phytochemicals in supplement form can replace the benefits gained from eating whole foods. That is, by eating *real food*!

Consuming a variety of plant-based foods on a daily basis in an adequate amount can reduce the oxidative stress and low-grade inflammatory markers. I recommend nine to twelve servings a day to gain these benefits.

MACRONUTRIENTS

Macronutrients also play a significant role in reducing inflammation and impacting metabolic health collectively:

» **INCREASE** your intake of vegetables, leafy greens, whole grains, fruits, nuts, fish, and olive oil.

» **DECREASE** your intake of processed meat, sugary drinks, processed foods, and saturated fat.

» **FATS:** The amount and type of fats included in the diet influence the degree of inflammation. PUFAs reduce the risk of heart disease due to their anti-inflammatory potential. In contrast, the increased consumption of saturated fats stimulate inflammatory transcription factor (NF-κβ), resulting in the synthesis of pro-inflammatory cytokines.

» **PROTEIN:** Studies have found that meat with a high fat content is more pro-inflammatory compared to lean meat. Proteins of plant origin and white meats decrease low-grade inflammation and help prevent chronic disease.

» **CARBOHYDRATES:** There is an inverse association between the intake of whole-grain carbohydrates and low-grade inflammation. The WHO recommends reducing sugar intake to less than 10 percent of total calories. Balanced macronutrient intake is important.

Typically, a good rule of thumb is 45 to 65 percent carbohydrates, 20 to 35 percent fats, and 25 to 30 percent protein.

Start the day with a good portion of protein to create satiety throughout the day. Many of the breakfast recipes make that seamless for you. They are also well balanced with good fats and carbohydrates that are high in fiber and resistant starches for detoxification and gut health benefits!

MICRONUTRIENTS

Without micronutrients, our cells can't function. We can't detox. We have no mitochondrial support and energy for our cells. Remember, nutrients (vitamins) are the fuel needed to keep the cells healthy and operating, leading to that next step of development or allowing for communication between cells of different organ systems.

Micronutrients are important as cofactors in metabolism, as they are involved in modulating enzymes and carrying out complex biochemical reactions. They are important for energy development, protein development, and DNA repair. Antioxidant potential is also another unique attribute. We know that reactive oxygen species, or "free radicals," have the potential to cause oxidative damage to our DNA. Now many people think antioxidants as only phytonutrients, but many vitamins serve as antioxidants, such as vitamins A and E. Overall, micronutrients play a central role in metabolism and in the maintenance of tissue function. So, consuming an adequate amount is vital.

The best way to get those micronutrients is through whole foods and a well-balanced diet as opposed to taking vitamins and supplements, as we don't see the same impact and clinical response from supplementation. The recipes in this book focus on a balance of micronutrients through fruits, vegetables, oils, seeds, nuts, herbs, and proteins to get you well-rounded nutrient support, so you don't have to think about it!

FIBER

Dietary fiber supports a healthy gut microbiota, physical barrier function, and immunity. It reduces the risk of developing many chronic, inflammatory diseases, such as Crohn's disease, type 2 diabetes, non-fatty liver disease, and chronic kidney disease. The microbiota includes bacteria, fungi, parasites, and viruses, and it can become imbalanced by a poor diet and other factors.

Dietary fiber is fermented by anaerobic bacteria in the large intestine to produce short-chain fatty acids (SCFAs), which reduce intestinal pH levels and inhibit pathogens. It helps ensure tight junctions and mucus production to prevent the transfer of intestinal bacteria and antigens across the epithelium. Dietary fiber also increases intestinal T regulatory cells and the production of immunoglobulin A (IgA) to reduce inflammation and microbial epithelial attachment.

Dietary fiber protects the liver by reducing the translocation of gut bacteria and inflammatory metabolites. Gut dysbiosis and increased intestinal permeability have been associated with liver damage due to raising the hepatic toxic load, thus burdening the immune system. A recent study confirmed that altered mucosal microbiota in cirrhotic patients stimulated an enhanced inflammatory response by hepatic cells. Dietary fiber also protects the liver from metabolic insults by slowing a rise in blood sugar/insulin. SCFAs have been found to reduce the need for hepatic glucose production and enhance insulin sensitivity. Increased dietary fiber intake has been shown to decrease blood LDL, BMI, and insulin resistance, leading to lower risk for type 2 diabetes.

Fiber sourced from whole food appears to be more beneficial than commercial fiber preparations. An apple, for example, yields beneficial compounds outside of its fiber, including magnesium, potassium, carotene, vitamin A, lutein, and phytosterols. A recent study also showed that fermentation of apple pectin gives rise to more diverse bacteria than that of inulin. That's just one example of a whole food and the many benefits it contains. As you can see, fiber is incredibly important to our immune and metabolic health, and you will find fiber in every recipe!

DETOXIFICATION

I always hear people say, "I feel like I need to detox my body." Is there any truth to that? Actually, yes!

Detoxification is the process by which the body eliminates harmful substances. We are dependent on our detox pathways to break down and eliminate toxic substances from our body. The majority of detoxification takes place within the liver, and supporting this process is key for maintaining health. Phase I and phase II detoxification pathways are responsible for breaking down and eliminating toxins that come from drugs, heavy metals, chemicals, diet, the environment, smoking, and poor nutrition. Some factors that affect detox pathways include smoking, medication or drug use, poor nutrition, and a polluted environment. While phase I reactions are less dependent on diet, phase II reactions require a steady, replenishable source of cofactors that come from a diet rich in phytonutrients, high-quality protein, vitamins, and fiber.

A diet lacking in these cofactors may cause buildup of highly toxic compounds from phase I reactions. Phase I uses enzymes from our liver to break down the toxins and send them to phase II to be removed. These enzymes break down toxic substances, but when they do, they are often more toxic than the original substance. These are called metabolites, and they can be harmful. Phase II needs cofactors that are found in whole foods to eliminate the toxins from phase I. Without these cofactors you can get a buildup of toxic substances in the body. Balance between the two phases is crucial to ensure toxins are eliminated efficiently.

A healthy diet and lifestyle are simple, easy ways to help maintain balance between the two detox pathways. That's why I always recommend eating nine to twelve servings of fruits and vegetables across the rainbow of colors, as well as other plant-based foods.

Research shows that a vegetarian diet lowers the risk of developing chronic diseases—and this may be in part due to their function in the body's detoxification pathways. Now I am not saying we should all be vegetarian. The important takeaway is that plants help support these detox pathways. You don't have to *only* consume plants, but you should consume a plentiful amount as part of a well-balanced diet. To make this easy and flexible, the recipes throughout the book include animal protein as well as substitutions using plant-based proteins.

AUTOIMMUNE OR METABOLIC CONDITIONS: HOW THESE RECIPES WORK

Ultimately, the goal with any autoimmune or metabolic condition is to:

1. Reduce inflammation
2. Optimize nutrition
3. Focus on your gut
4. Manage stress and sleep

REDUCE INFLAMMATION

We focus so much on how inflammation is a BAD thing, and we forget that the inflammatory response is to help you heal. It's chronic inflammation that is damaging; a response that doesn't go away and is constantly lingering in the body is associated with arthritis, cancer, diabetes, and autoimmune disease. Typical symptoms associated with chronic inflammation include body pain, constant fatigue, gut disorders, and frequent infections.

Controlling chronic inflammation starts with removing inflammatory foods:

» Simple sugars and refined and processed white flour promote bacterial overgrowth and lead to leaky gut.

» High-sugar foods cause immunosuppression for 2 to 4 hours after eating.

» Saturated fats that are high in omega-6 fatty acids are inflammatory.

» Food allergens can form immune complexes and lead to inflammation.

» Gluten is the biggest perpetuator of leaky gut. Gliadin is the toxic, immunogenic component of gluten, and it is mediated by T cell activation. When gliadin interacts with the intestinal epithelium, it increases leaky gut.

» The three proteins in dairy—lactose, casein, and whey—can all cause inflammation in different individuals.

OPTIMIZE NUTRITION

Instead of focusing on specific fruits or vegetables, make a goal to consume nine servings of plant-based foods daily. Make it a *variety* of colors and types. Eat the rainbow, and this will ensure you are getting adequate nutrients that work in synergy. Keep inflammation down and avoid foods that cause or aggravate inflammation.

FOCUS ON GUT HEALTH

The bacteria in your gut affect more than just your belly. When you have a balance, your immune system is strong, you have good digestion, your skin glows, and your mood is improved! Consume adequate amounts of fiber to help produce SCFAs, which feed good bacteria and help ensure a balanced gut microbiota.

start with 10 minutes

The best way to start exercising is to start! If you've been sedentary, start by walking for 10 minutes and build up to about 30 minutes. A recent study found that even 20 minutes on the treadmill—and not at breakneck speed—reduced inflammation!

Listen to your body and find a type of exercise that works for you. My advice to anyone is do something you ENJOY. If you enjoy it, you will stick with it!

MANAGE STRESS AND SLEEP

Stress has been shown to be associated with disease onset and the exacerbation of rheumatoid arthritis, systemic lupus erythematous, inflammatory bowel disease, multiple sclerosis, Graves' disease, Hashimoto's, and other autoimmune conditions.

For example, the role of stress in the pathophysiology of thyroid autoimmune disease involves the immune system and the effects of the various hormones secreted during episodes of stress. During stress, the secretion of thyrotropin is suppressed and thyrotrophic-releasing hormone action is blunted. Moreover, the activation of thyroid hormone in peripheral tissue is decreased during stress.

High anxiety levels as a result of stress increase inflammatory cytokines TNF-alpha and IL-6. TNF-alpha is a cytokine that mimics melatonin, a hormone responsible for the circadian rhythms of different physiological functions. Our melatonin peaks when our cortisol is at its lowest—so cortisol and melatonin are a balance scale. Melatonin decreases the production of pro-inflammatory cytokines and exerts an anti-inflammatory effect. But under stress our cortisol is elevated, which means melatonin is low and therefore we are in an inflammatory state.

It's important to be mindful of stress and how to manage it. Psychological therapy and cognitive behavioral therapy aimed to reduce stress levels are effective in influencing better outcomes in many autoimmune diseases. Sleep has an important role to play in the human immune system and is critical in the restoration and maintenance of homeostasis. Sleep deprivation has a profound impact on health, well-being, and the ability to resist infection. Sleep disorders may trigger immune system abnormalities, inducing auto-antibody production and possibly leading to the development of autoimmune disease.

SO WHERE DO WE BEGIN?

Maybe you are searching for how to achieve optimal health. Maybe you are looking to prevent disease. Maybe you just want to know more about your own nutrition. I firmly believe that if you understand "the why" behind a concept, then you are more likely to adopt it, practice it, and preach it! So read and reread these foundational chapters, as needed.

Health is not one size fits all; we are all unique in our own way, and our genetics are a big component of that. Our lifestyle, exposure to toxins, and diet all influence our genes to turn disease on or off. Being in a pro-inflammatory state negatively affects our immune system and disrupts our metabolic health, leading to disease development. We can reverse this process and quench that inflammatory response by increasing phytonutrients in our diet.

If you are recently diagnosed with an autoimmune or a metabolic disease, or you have unexplainable symptoms and you're looking for answers, it's completely normal to feel absolutely lost and confused and maybe even helpless. That's okay! Nutrition is more than half the battle, so you are in the right place to tackle your health and start feeling your best. Recognizing how we can prevent disease or reduce unexplained symptoms starts with our lifestyle, our environment, and our nutrition.

This book makes it simple for you to consume nutrient-dense, phytonutrient-diverse, macronutrient-balanced, real, whole food recipes! These specific nutrients are necessary for cellular optimization. Some of these nutrients include curcumin, flavonoids, omega-3 fatty acids (PUFAs), organosulfur compounds, antioxidants (vitamins C and E, grapeseed extract), and the brassica vegetables (Brussels sprouts, broccoli, cauliflower).

Rather than giving you a prescribed diet to follow, I have taken the top 100 foods to reduce inflammation, nourish your gut, aid detoxification, and increase antioxidant potential from *Immunity Food Fix* and put them in nourishing recipes you can enjoy! Just keep in mind that variety matters. Consume nine to twelve servings of plant-based foods per day in a variety of colors and types, such as nuts, seeds, herbs, and healthy fats. The recipes in this book will get you to that goal, if not beyond! They were thoughtfully created to support all the concepts covered in these chapters. So you don't have to do the thinking, you just have to do the eating!

Throughout this book, you will find recipes for snacks, drinks, breakfast, lunch, dinner, and dessert! Many of these recipes can be made in batches and eaten throughout the week to ensure you are eating a healthy diet and avoiding inflammatory foods. Each recipe combines healthy oils, herbs, seeds, nuts, fruits, and vegetables, giving you that variety of phytonutrients, micronutrients, and macronutrients you need for a well-balanced diet. The nutrient variety in each recipe supports digestion, satiety, metabolic health, and immune health.

What are you waiting for? Get your immunity food fix on—and start cooking!

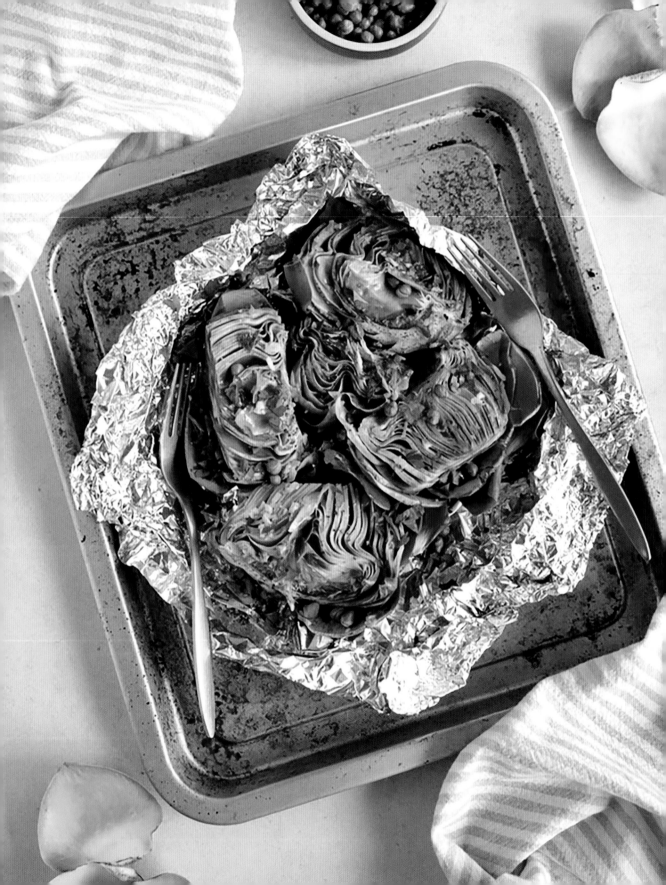

CHAPTER FIVE

SNACKS, APPETIZERS & LITTLE BITES

Snacks are always top of mind, whether it's to take on the go or because so many of us are working from home and running to our pantry for options. Sometimes mindless snacking leaves us with empty calories, glucose dysregulation, and a feeling of never being satisfied. This can really throw us off track when trying to get our immunity food fix!

The dips found in this chapter, such as the Roasted Eggplant Dip (page 59) or the Beet Hummus (page 60), are a great way to enjoy whole foods, reduce inflammation, and boost nutrition. Nutritious nuts are always a great snack option, especially when you're on the go. They are high in good fats and protein. But why not spice it up by trying the Curry Roasted Almonds, Cashews, and Walnuts (page 70)? So easy, yet so satisfying!

These recipes are bursting with flavor, immune-boosting properties, and antioxidant potential, and they make for excellent little bites. Whether you are looking for a delicious dip, a fun side salad, an immunity-boosting soup, or a batch of muffins you can whip up, this chapter has it all!

Find your side: simple, satisfying, and immune supporting!

Roasted Globe Artichokes with Garlic
and Lemon, page 64

tomato-peach fruit salsa

with black beans and lime

SERVINGS: 12
PREP TIME: 10 MIN
COOK TIME: 0 MIN

VEGETARIAN
VEGAN
DAIRY-FREE
GLUTEN-FREE
GRAIN-FREE

superfoods used

OLIVE OIL
LIME
BASIL
TOMATO
PEACH
AVOCADO

nutrition info

CALORIES: 224
FAT: 5
CARBS: 9
NET CARBS: 6
FIBER: 3
PROTEIN: 3

This salsa is a fantastic, satiating snack. The black beans increase protein and fiber in this recipe, and the addition of olive oil helps your body absorb the vitamins. The synergies of the tomato and peach add vitamins A and C, which bring antioxidant and anti-inflammatory benefits as they dance around in your stomach. This is delicious served over a bed of greens or over warm brown rice or quinoa!

SALSA

- 3 tablespoons (45 ml) olive oil
- Zest from ½ medium (11 g) fresh lime
- 2 tablespoons (30 ml) fresh lime juice
- 1 tablespoon (15 ml) raw apple cider vinegar
- 1 teaspoon (6 g) sea salt
- ½ teaspoon (3 g) black pepper
- ¼ cup (4 g) fresh cilantro, minced
- 2 tablespoons (2 g) fresh basil, minced
- 1 medium (15 g) scallion, minced
- ½ cups (300 g) cherry tomatoes, halved
- 1 medium (150 g) fresh peach, pitted and diced
- 1 medium (150 g) avocado, peeled, pitted, and diced
- 15 ounces (425 g) cooked black beans, rinsed
- Honey
- Gluten-free crackers or chips

To make the salsa, add the olive oil to a mixing bowl, followed by the lime zest and juice, vinegar, salt, pepper, cilantro, basil, and scallion. Mix well.

Add the tomatoes, peach, avocado, and black beans. Gently toss until everything is coated in the mixture. Drizzle honey (to taste) over the salsa, and toss it one more time.

Serve with your favorite crackers or chips. Store any leftovers in the fridge in an airtight container for up to 3 days.

cantaloupe and smoked salmon caprese

with lemon-mint pesto

SERVINGS: 6
PREP TIME: 10 MIN
COOK TIME: 0 MIN

DAIRY-FREE
GLUTEN-FREE
GRAIN-FREE
(VEGAN OPTION)

Cantaloupe is rich in vitamin C, which helps our immune system. It is also a good source of vitamin B6, dietary fiber, folate, niacin, and potassium, which help maintain healthy blood sugar levels and metabolism. Smoked salmon, one of the best sources of omega-3 fatty acids, is linked to decreased inflammation, specifically reducing markers TNF-a and IL-6. The pesto is delicious and adds so many immunity benefits. Basil contains a variety of antioxidants, protecting our cells from damage. Lemons give this process an added bonus because of the flavonoids hesperidin and hesperetin; both provide a robust antioxidant profile and more vitamin C!

superfoods used

CANTALOUPE
BASIL
OLIVE OIL
LEMON
GARLIC
PEPPERMINT
WALNUT
SALMON

LEMON-MINT PESTO

- ¼ cup (60 ml) olive oil
- 2 tablespoons (30 ml) fresh lemon juice
- ½ teaspoon (3 g) sea salt
- 2 tablespoons (10 g) nutritional yeast
- 1 small (4 g) clove garlic, minced
- 1 cup (20 g) fresh basil
- 2 cups (50 g) fresh mint
- ¼ cup (28 g) walnuts

SALAD

- 1 cup (200 g) sliced tomato
- 6 ounces (170 g) smoked salmon, torn into pieces (omit for vegan option)
- Handful of fresh basil
- 2 cups (312 g) chopped fresh cantaloupe

To make the pesto, add the olive oil, lemon juice, salt, nutritional yeast, and garlic to a food processor. Pulse a few times until everything is well combined. Add the basil, mint, and walnuts (in batches if necessary). Continue to pulse until creamy.

To make the salad, stack the tomato slices, salmon, and basil leaves on top of the cantaloupe pieces. Secure with a toothpick. Repeat until you have used all the cantaloupe, salmon, and basil.

Serve with the pesto. Store any leftovers in the fridge in an airtight container for up to 2 days.

nutrition info

CALORIES: 235
FAT: 17
CARBS: 8
NET CARBS: 4
FIBER: 4
PROTEIN: 16

nutrition info for vegan option

CALORIES: 147
FAT: 13
CARBS: 7
NET CARBS: 3
FIBER: 4
PROTEIN: 3

watermelon, cucumber, and red pepper salad

with mint and basil

VEGAN
VEGETARIAN
DAIRY-FREE
GLUTEN-FREE
GRAIN-FREE

superfoods used

OLIVE OIL
LIME
BASIL
PEPPERMINT
WATERMELON
CUCUMBER
RED BELL PEPPER
HEMP SEED

nutrition info

CALORIES: 69
FAT: 4
CARBS: 8
NET CARBS: 7
FIBER: 1
PROTEIN: 1

This salad is rich in lycopene, aiding in the body's detoxification of free radicals that affect our health at a cellular level. Combining three different red foods—watermelon, tomato, and red pepper—really gives that detox boost! Red peppers are also a great source of fiber, which is essential for detoxification and critical to helping gut microbes flourish. Throwing in some green cucumber provides an anti-inflammatory and immune-boosting benefit.

SALAD

- 2 tablespoons (30 ml) olive oil
- 2 tablespoons (30 ml) red wine vinegar
- Zest from ½ medium (11 g) fresh lime
- 2 tablespoons (30 ml) fresh lime juice
- 1 teaspoon (6 g) sea salt
- ½ teaspoon (3 g) black pepper
- 2 tablespoons (2 g) fresh basil, minced
- 10 fresh peppermint leaves, minced
- 4 cups (610 g) cubed fresh watermelon
- 1 large (301 g) cucumber, halved, seeded, and diced
- 1 large (165 g) red bell pepper, cored, seeded, and chopped

GARNISH

- 1 tablespoon (10 g) hemp seeds

To make the salad, add the olive oil, red wine vinegar, lime zest and juice, salt, pepper, basil, and mint to a mixing bowl. Stir to combine. Add the watermelon, cucumber, and red bell pepper. Gently toss until everything is coated.

Serve garnished with hemp seeds. Store any leftovers in the fridge in an airtight container for up to 3 days.

roasted butternut and avocado salad

with lemon and kalamata olives

SERVINGS: 8
PREP TIME: 10 MIN
COOK TIME: 30 MIN

VEGAN
VEGETARIAN
DAIRY-FREE
GLUTEN-FREE
GRAIN-FREE

Savory, roasted vegetable salads make an excellent snack option. With its bright orange color, butternut squash is high in carotenoids and a great source of vitamin A, which is vital for our immune system. Avocado and kalamata olives are a great source of healthy fats and fiber. This salad is wonderful served in a bowl with a fork, or try it smashed over a piece of gluten-free toast!

superfoods used

AVOCADO OIL
LIME
BASIL
THYME
SAGE
ROSEMARY
BUTTERNUT SQUASH
AVOCADO

SALAD

- 2 tablespoons (30 ml) avocado oil
- Zest from ½ medium (13 g) fresh lemon
- 2 tablespoons (30 ml) fresh lemon juice
- 1 teaspoon (6 g) sea salt
- ½ teaspoon (3 g) black pepper
- 2 teaspoons (4 g) dried Italian seasoning or a mixture of dried basil, oregano, thyme, sage, and rosemary
- 4 cups (820 g) cubed butternut squash
- 1 medium (40 g) shallot, minced
- ¼ cup (4 g) fresh parsley, minced
- 2 medium (300 g) avocados, peeled and diced
- 10 (30 g) pitted kalamata olives, chopped

nutrition info

CALORIES: 132
FAT: 10
CARBS: 9
NET CARBS: 4
FIBER: 5
PROTEIN: 2

Preheat the oven to 400°F (200°C). Line a baking sheet with parchment paper.

To make the salad, add the oil to a large mixing bowl, followed by the lemon zest and juice, salt, pepper, and Italian seasoning.

Gently toss the butternut and shallot in the oil mixture until it is coated. Arrange on the prepared baking sheet and bake in the oven for 30 minutes, tossing at the halfway mark.

Remove from the oven and transfer to a mixing bowl. Add the parsley, avocado, and kalamata olives to the bowl. Gently toss with the butternut.

Serve and enjoy! Store any leftovers in the fridge in an airtight container for up to 3 days.

sweet grilled peaches and apricots

with basil and walnuts

SERVINGS: 8
PREP TIME: 5 MIN
COOK TIME: 10 MIN

VEGETARIAN
VEGAN
DAIRY-FREE
GLUTEN-FREE
GRAIN-FREE

superfoods used

AVOCADO OIL
LEMON
CINNAMON
PEACH
APRICOT
BASIL
WALNUT

nutrition info

CALORIES: 76
FAT: 5
CARBS: 8
NET CARBS: 7
FIBER: 1
PROTEIN: 1

Grilling fruit is a wonderful way to prepare the season's finest offerings as grilling caramelizes the sugars and brings out its naturally sweet flavors. When selecting your peaches and apricots for this recipe, the riper the better, as the antioxidant count goes up. The skin of the peach and the pulp of the apricot contain the best nutrients, so it's important to consume the entire fruit for the benefit. This recipe pairs sweet with savory, and it is a fantastic appetizer for a social gathering or as a side to your weekly dinner menu.

FRUIT

- 2 tablespoons (30 ml) avocado oil
- Zest from ½ medium (13 g) fresh lemon
- 1 tablespoon (15 ml) fresh lemon juice
- 1 teaspoon (6 g) sea salt
- ½ teaspoon (3 g) black pepper
- ½ teaspoon (2 g) ground cinnamon
- 2 medium (300 g) ripe peaches, halved and pitted
- 4 medium (140 g) ripe apricots, halved and pitted

GARNISH

- 1 tablespoon (15 g) honey or maple syrup
- 2 tablespoons (2 g) fresh basil, minced
- ¼ cup (28 g) chopped walnuts

To prepare the fruit, add the oil, lemon zest and juice, salt, pepper, and cinnamon to a mixing bowl. Stir to combine. Brush the peaches and apricots with the oil mixture until they are fully coated.

Preheat a grill pan (or outdoor grill) over high heat. When hot, place the fruit on the grill, cut-side down. Cook for 3 minutes per side. Do not move once on the pan, except to flip them, so that the fruits get distinct grill lines.

Serve garnished with the honey, basil, and walnuts. Store any leftovers in the fridge in an airtight container for up to 5 days.

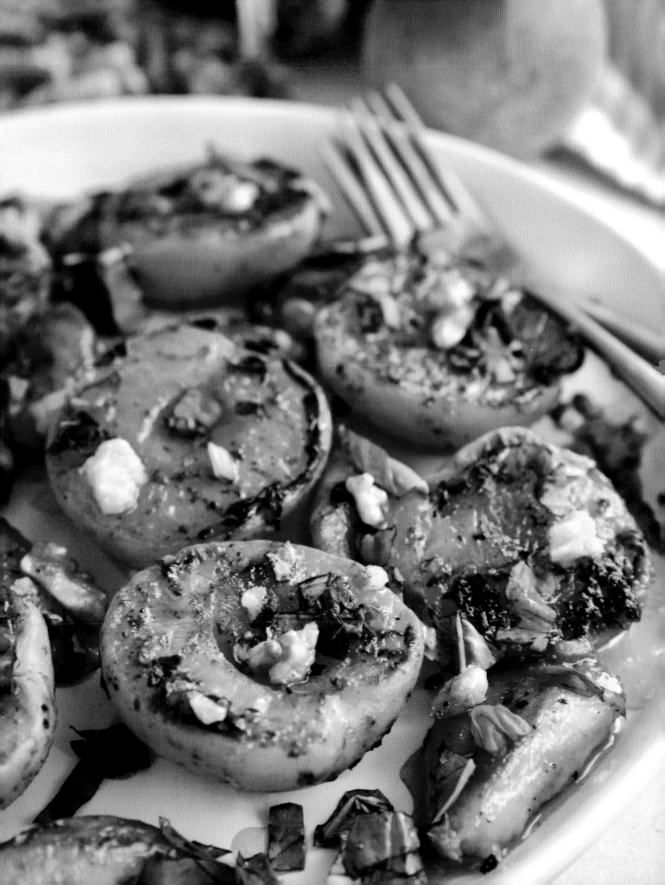

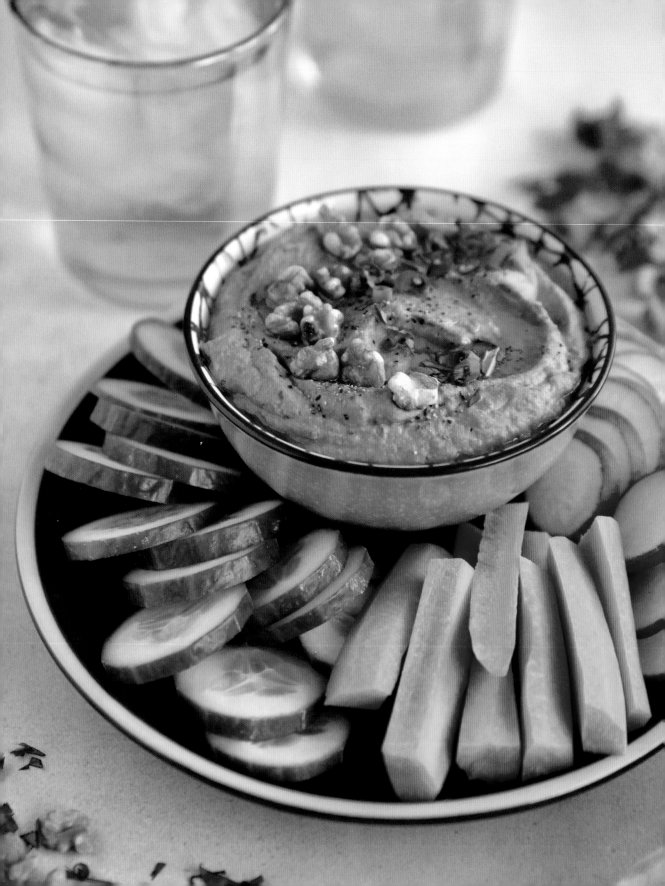

roasted eggplant dip

with lemon and toasted walnuts

SERVINGS: 8
PREP TIME: 10 MIN
COOK TIME: 45 MIN

VEGAN
VEGETARIAN
DAIRY-FREE
GLUTEN-FREE
GRAIN-FREE

Eggplant is rich in fiber and antioxidants, and it also contains inositol, which has a positive impact on the body's ability to control blood sugar. You can use any toasted nut or seed in this recipe; try it with toasted almonds, pine nuts, or sunflower seeds! Seeds are a powerhouse of nutrition, giving this dish added omega-3 fatty acids, protein, and fiber. This dish can be served at room temperature, or enjoy it chilled out of the fridge.

superfoods used

OLIVE OIL
EGGPLANT
LEMON
SESAME SEED
WALNUT

EGGPLANT DIP

- 1 medium (548 g) eggplant, halved
- ¼ cup (28 g) chopped walnuts, toasted
- 2 tablespoons (30 ml) olive oil
- Zest from ½ medium (13 g) fresh lemon
- 2 tablespoons (30 ml) fresh lemon juice
- ¼ cup (60 g) tahini
- 2 small (8 g) cloves garlic, minced
- 1 teaspoon (6 g) sea salt
- ½ teaspoon (3 g) black pepper

GARNISH

- 1 tablespoon (15 ml) olive oil
- 2 tablespoons (14 g) chopped walnuts, toasted
- Sprinkle of black pepper
- ¼ cup (4 g) fresh cilantro, minced
- 1 medium (15 g) scallion, minced

Preheat the oven to 400°F (200°C). Line a baking sheet with parchment paper.

To make the eggplant dip, place the eggplant halves face down on the prepared baking sheet. Roast until it is very soft and the skin is wrinkly, about 45 minutes. Remove from the oven and allow to cool to room temperature.

In a food processor, pulse the walnuts until fine and crumbly. Add the olive oil, lemon zest and juice, tahini, and garlic. Pulse together well. Add the flesh of the eggplant and season with salt and pepper. Pulse until very creamy, scraping down the sides of the bowl as needed.

Transfer to a serving bowl. Garnish with the olive oil, toasted walnuts, pepper, cilantro, and scallion.

Serve and enjoy! Store any leftovers in the fridge in an airtight container for up to 5 days.

nutrition info

CALORIES: 127
FAT: 11
CARBS: 7
NET CARBS: 4
FIBER: 3
PROTEIN: 2

beet hummus

with carrot and jicama sticks

SERVINGS: 12
PREP TIME: 15 MIN
COOK TIME: 40 MIN

VEGAN
VEGETARIAN
DAIRY-FREE
GLUTEN-FREE
GRAIN-FREE

superfoods used

BEET
OLIVE OIL
GARLIC
CHICKPEA
LEMON
SESAME SEED
CARROT
JICAMA

nutrition info

CALORIES: 199
FAT: 11
CARBS: 21
NET CARBS: 15
FIBER: 6
PROTEIN: 6

This recipe is packed with vitamins and nutrients from root vegetables. Beets are bursting with antioxidants and betalains, which have excellent anti-inflammatory action. Carrots are high in beta-carotene and also help balance hormones in the body. Jicama is a wonderful prebiotic, aiding in digestion and also excellent at regulating blood sugar levels. This recipe combines restoring roots in a variety of colors to gain that immunomodulatory and anti-inflammatory benefit. Serve this at a gathering or enjoy it throughout the week!

BEET HUMMUS

- 3 cups (400 g) peeled and chopped beetroot
- ¼ cup (60 ml) olive oil, divided
- 2 small (8 g) cloves garlic, minced
- 1½ teaspoons (9 g) sea salt, divided
- ½ teaspoon (3 g) black pepper
- 1 teaspoon (5 g) ground cumin
- 3 cups (510 g) cooked chickpeas, drained
- Zest from ½ medium (13 g) fresh lemon
- 3 tablespoons (45 ml) fresh lemon juice
- ⅓ cup (90 g) tahini

Preheat the oven to 400°F (200°C). Line a baking sheet with parchment paper.

To make the beet hummus, add the beets, 2 tablespoons (30 ml) of the olive oil, garlic, 1 teaspoon (6 g) of the salt, pepper, and cumin to a mixing bowl. Toss together well.

Arrange the beets on the prepared baking sheet and roast until very soft, 35 to 40 minutes, tossing at the halfway mark. Remove from the oven and allow to cool to room temperature.

Transfer the beets to a food processor. Pulse until very creamy, scraping down the sides as needed. Add the remaining 2 tablespoons (30 ml) olive oil, remaining ½ teaspoon salt, chickpeas, lemon zest and juice, and tahini. Pulse together well until very creamy, scraping down the sides of the bowl as needed.

Transfer to a serving bowl. Garnish with the olive oil, sesame seeds, and cilantro. Serve with the sliced carrot and jicama.

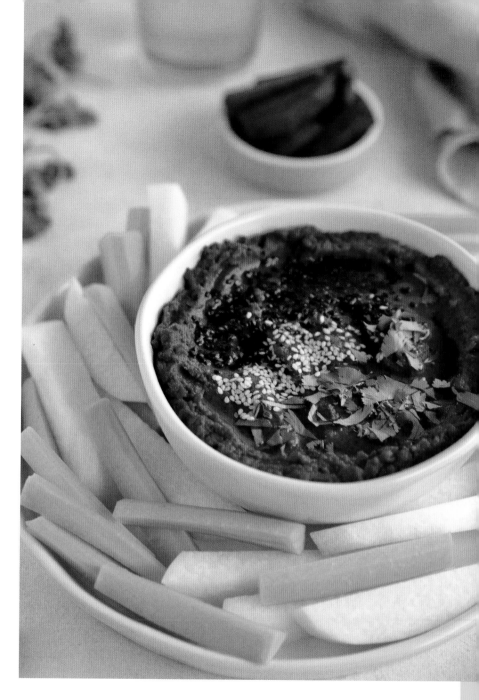

GARNISH

- 1 tablespoon (15 ml) olive oil

- 1 tablespoon (10 g) black or white sesame seeds

- ¼ cup (4 g) fresh cilantro or parsley, minced

CARROTS AND JICAMA

- 4 medium (240 g) carrots, peeled and cut into sticks

- ½ medium (350 g) jicama, peeled and cut into sticks

Serve and enjoy! Store any leftovers in the fridge in an airtight container for up to 5 days.

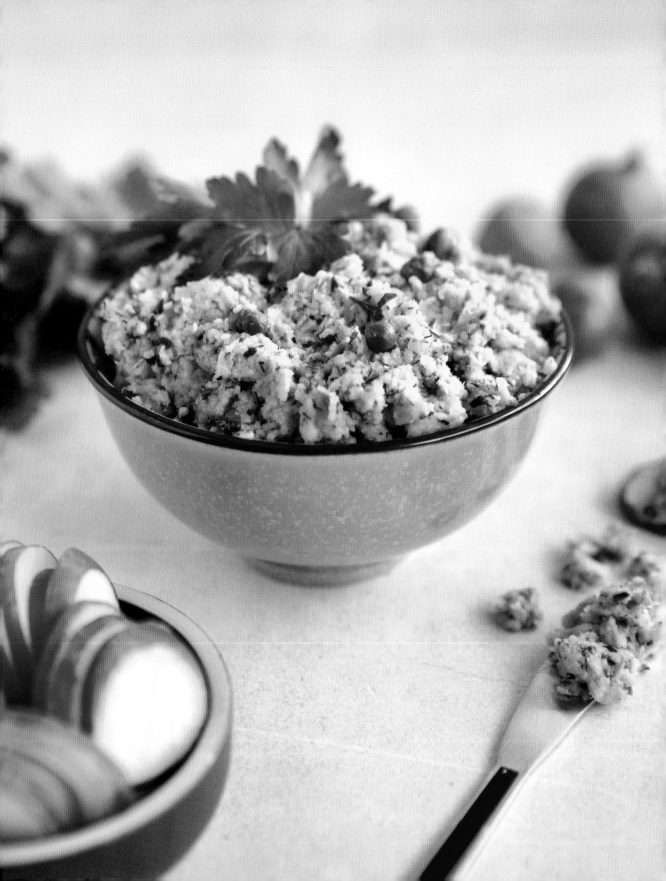

smoked trout dip

Smoked trout is rich in protein and omega-3 fatty acids. It supports heart and brain health. The combination of garlic and tahini takes this dip to the next level. Tahini is a paste made from ground sesame seeds. Sesame seeds contain the lignan sesamin, which has anti-inflammatory activities, blocking the release of pro-inflammatory cytokines. Pair this delicious savory dip with your favorite veggie crudités, such as carrot, celery, cucumber, and radish. It's also delicious served over a bed of greens or with your favorite gluten-free crackers.

SERVINGS: 6
PREP TIME: 10 MIN
COOK TIME: 0 MIN

DAIRY-FREE
GLUTEN-FREE
GRAIN-FREE

superfoods used

OLIVE OIL
LEMON
SESAME SEED
HEMP SEED

nutrition info

CALORIES: 221
FAT: 20
CARBS: 4
NET CARBS: 3
FIBER: 1
PROTEIN: 9

SMOKED TROUT DIP

- ¼ cup (60 ml) olive oil
- Zest from ½ medium (13 g) fresh lemon
- 2 tablespoons (30 ml) fresh lemon juice
- ¼ cup (60 g) tahini
- 1 small (4 g) clove garlic, minced
- 1 teaspoon (6 g) sea salt
- ½ teaspoon (3 g) black pepper
- ½ cup (8 g) fresh parsley, chopped
- 1 tablespoon (1 g) fresh dill
- 2 tablespoons (14 g) capers, drained
- 6 ounces (170 g) smoked trout, skin removed

GARNISH

- 1 tablespoon (15 ml) olive oil
- 1 tablespoon (10 g) hemp seeds
- 1 tablespoon (1 g) fresh parsley, chopped

To make the dip, in a food processor, add the olive oil, lemon zest and juice, tahini, garlic, salt, and pepper and pulse until creamy and well combined. Add the parsley, dill, capers, and smoked trout. Pulse several times until thoroughly mixed but leaving some of its texture (not a complete puree).

Transfer to a serving bowl. Garnish with the olive oil, hemp seeds, and parsley.

Serve and enjoy! Store any leftovers in the fridge in an airtight container for up to 2 days.

roasted globe artichokes with garlic and lemon

SERVINGS: 6
PREP TIME: 10 MIN
COOK TIME: 40 MIN

DAIRY-FREE
GLUTEN-FREE
GRAIN-FREE
VEGAN
VEGETARIAN

Artichokes are a great source of prebiotic inulin, which is food for our gut microbiome. They also are rich in fiber and support liver health by increasing bile flow. Their health benefits are worth the effort of trimming and cooking, and they are absolutely delicious. The garlic in this recipe brings the immunomodulatory properties from the active ingredient allicin. What's critical in this recipe is to make sure you crush the garlic first to activate the process before roasting to gain those benefits.

superfoods used

**GLOBE ARTICHOKES
AVOCADO OIL
LEMON
ONION
GARLIC**

nutrition info

CALORIES: 167
FAT: 14
CARBS: 10
NET CARBS: 5
FIBER: 5
PROTEIN: 3

GLOBE ARTICHOKES

- 3 large (450 g) globe artichokes
- 2 tablespoons (30 ml) fresh lemon juice
- Zest from 1 (26 g) fresh lemon
- 6 tablespoons (90 ml) avocado oil
- 2 teaspoons (12 g) sea salt
- 1 teaspoon (6 g) black pepper
- 1 medium (40 g) shallot, minced
- 4 small (16 g) cloves garlic, minced

GARNISH

- ½ cup (8 g) fresh parsley, chopped
- 2 tablespoons (14 g) capers, drained
- Fresh lemon wedges

Preheat the oven to 400°F (200°C).

To prepare the artichokes, cut off the stems. With your hands, then remove the tough outer leaves until you have reached the softer leaves. Using a serrated knife, cut off the top 1 inch (2.5 cm) and discard. Cut the artichokes in half lengthwise and remove the fuzzy middle choke from the inside. Squeeze fresh lemon juice all over the insides of the artichoke halves to prevent oxidation.

Place each artichoke half, cut-side up, on a piece of aluminum foil large enough to wrap around and secure, similar to a baked potato. Sprinkle over the lemon zest, drizzle with the oil, and season with the salt and pepper. Place shallot and garlic in each half and tightly secure with the foil. Bake in the oven for 35 to 40 minutes, or until soft.

Serve garnished with the parsley and capers and extra lemon wedges. Store any leftovers in the fridge in an airtight container for up to 5 days.

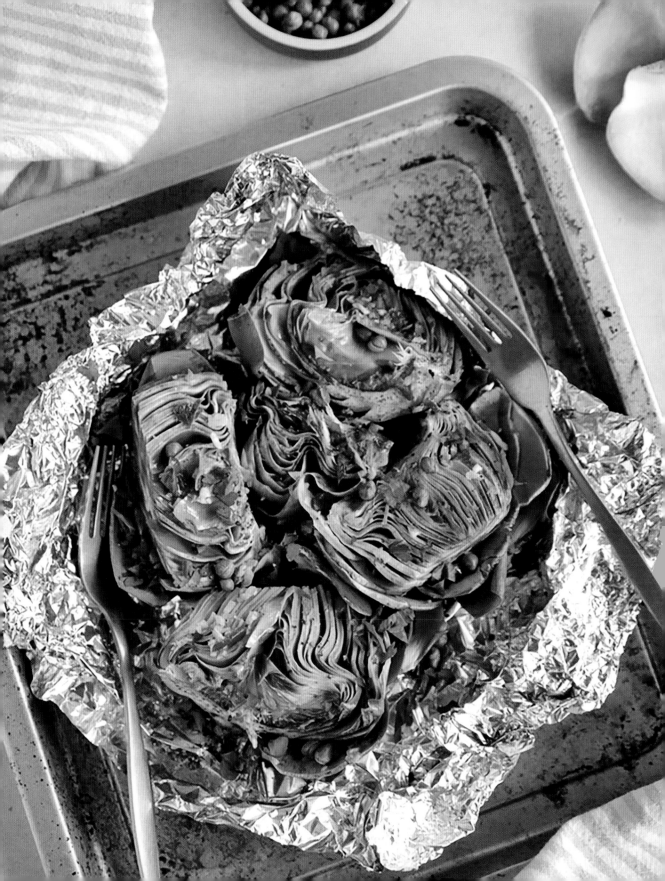

sweet potato sunchoke dip

SERVINGS: 8
PREP TIME: 10 MIN
COOK TIME: 45 MIN

VEGETARIAN
VEGAN
DAIRY-FREE
GLUTEN-FREE
GRAIN-FREE

superfoods used

SWEET POTATO
SUNCHOKE
(JERUSALEM
ARTICHOKE)
CHICKPEA
GARLIC
TURMERIC
OLIVE OIL
LEMON
SESAME SEED
HAZELNUT

nutrition info

CALORIES: 255
FAT: 16
CARBS: 23
NET CARBS: 17
FIBER: 6
PROTEIN: 7

Sunchokes (Jerusalem artichokes) are high in potassium, magnesium, iron, and calcium. They are wonderful at helping stabilize blood sugar. Combining these with restoring roots, such as sweet potato, garlic, and turmeric, gives this dish a true immunity boost. Sweet potatoes are super tasty, and they are a great starch to stabilize blood sugar as well. You get it all with this one—antioxidant, anti-inflammatory, and glucose-regulating benefits! You can find sunchokes in the produce section where roots, such as fresh ginger and turmeric, are sold.

SWEET POTATO SUNCHOKE DIP

- 1 medium (130 g) sweet potato, scrubbed clean
- 5 ounces (150 g) sunchokes (Jerusalem artichokes), scrubbed clean
- 15 ounces (425 g) chickpeas, rinsed
- 2 small (8 g) cloves garlic, minced
- 1 teaspoon (6 g) sea salt
- ½ teaspoon (3 g) black pepper
- 1 teaspoon (2 g) ground turmeric
- 1 teaspoon (3 g) dried red pepper flakes
- ¼ cup (60 ml) olive oil
- 2 tablespoons (30 ml) fresh lemon juice
- ¼ cup (60 g) tahini

GARNISH

- 1 tablespoon (15 ml) olive oil
- 2 tablespoons (16 g) chopped hazelnuts

  Sprinkle of black pepper
- ¼ cup (4 g) fresh parsley, minced

Preheat the oven to 375°F (190°C). Line a baking sheet with parchment paper.

To make the dip, poke the sweet potato with a fork several times and wrap it in aluminum foil. Do the same with the sunchokes. Arrange the wrapped vegetables on the prepared baking sheet, cover everything with aluminum foil, and bake in the oven until very soft, about 45 minutes. Remove from the oven and allow to cool to room temperature.

Remove the peels from the sweet potato and the sunchokes and discard. Transfer the flesh of the sweet potato and sunchokes to a food processor. Add the chickpeas, garlic, salt, pepper, turmeric, and red pepper flakes. Pulse until smooth.

Add the olive oil, lemon juice, and tahini, and pulse together well. Transfer to a serving bowl. Garnish with the olive oil, hazelnuts, pepper, and parsley.

Serve and enjoy! Store any leftovers in the fridge in an airtight container for up to 5 days.

savory mushroom and chestnut soup

SERVINGS: 8
PREP TIME: 10 MIN
COOK TIME: 30 MIN

DAIRY-FREE
GLUTEN-FREE
VEGAN
VEGETARIAN
GRAIN-FREE

Chestnuts are rich in gallic and ellagic antioxidants, which increase in concentration when cooked, so be assured you are getting maximum nutrition in this soup. They are also high in fiber, making them a great prebiotic and supporting gut health and digestion. The mushrooms help give this recipe an immunity boost with anti-inflammatory properties. Adding rosemary to this combination brings a deeper flavor to the soup, and it boosts the overall anti-inflammatory potential.

SOUP

- 2 tablespoons (30 ml) avocado oil
- 1 medium (150 g) yellow onion, chopped
- 2 small (8 g) cloves garlic, minced
- 1 teaspoon (6 g) sea salt
- ½ teaspoon (3 g) black pepper
- 2 cups (260 g) peeled and chopped chestnuts
- 4 cups (360 g) cremini mushrooms, chopped
- 1 tablespoon (3 g) dried rosemary
- 2 cups (480 ml) vegetable stock
- 1 can (14 ounces, or 400 ml) full-fat coconut milk
- 2 tablespoons (30 ml) coconut aminos

GARNISH

- ½ cup (120 g) reserved sautéed onion, garlic, chestnut, and mushrooms
- ¼ cup (4 g) fresh parsley, minced
- A few sprigs of fresh thyme

To make the soup, add the oil to a large pot over medium-low heat. Add the onion and garlic and season with the salt and pepper. Sauté until the onion is soft and has begun to brown, about 10 minutes.

Add the chestnuts and sauté for about 5 minutes, then add the mushrooms and rosemary. Sauté until the mushrooms are soft, about 5 minutes. Using a spoon, scoop about ½ cup (120 g) of the vegetable mixture out of the pot and set aside to use as garnish.

Add the vegetable stock, coconut milk, and coconut aminos and stir well. Decrease the heat to low and simmer for 10 minutes.

Turn off the heat and transfer to a blender. Blend on high speed until it is very creamy.

Serve the soup garnished with the reserved sautéed onion, parsley, and thyme. Store any leftovers in the fridge in an airtight container for up to 5 days.

superfoods used

AVOCADO OIL
ONION
GARLIC
MUSHROOM
CHESTNUT
ROSEMARY
THYME

nutrition info

CALORIES: 205
FAT: 16
CARBS: 12
NET CARBS: 11
FIBER: 1
PROTEIN: 3

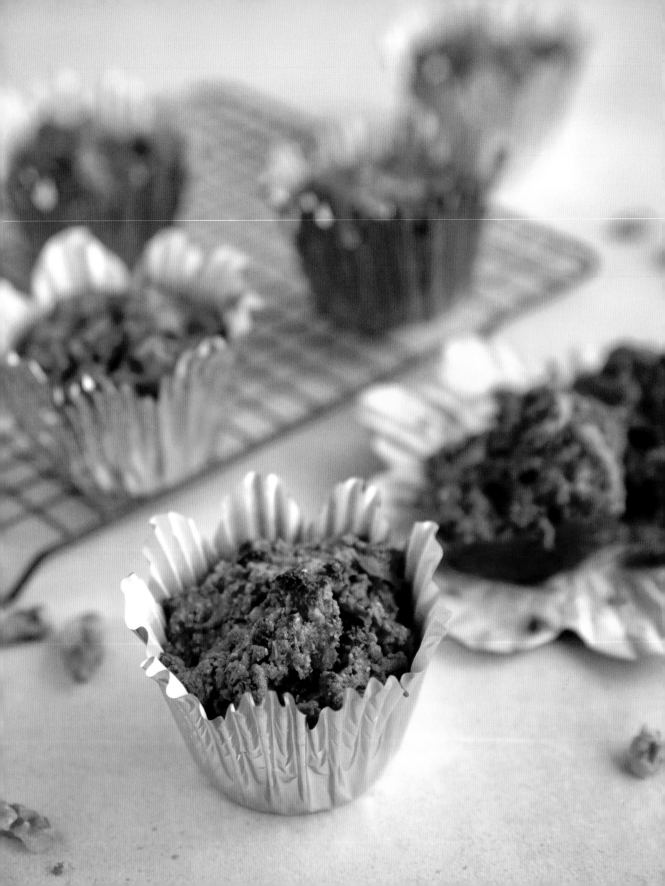

carrot-ginger spice spelt muffins

SERVINGS: 12
PREP TIME: 10 MIN
COOK TIME: 25 MIN

DAIRY-FREE
VEGETARIAN

These carrot spice muffins are a treat served with a cup of your favorite herbal tea. You may see an ingredient here you've never tried: spelt flour. Spelt flour is an ancient grain that is uniquely high in protein. While not gluten-free, it is easier to digest than traditional wheat and contains higher amounts of fiber. The added cinnamon in this recipe is excellent for glucose regulation. Try these sliced in half with melted coconut butter and some rooibos, or take along for a quick on-the-go breakfast!

superfoods used

CARROT
WALNUT
AVOCADO OIL
FLAXSEED
ALMOND
CINNAMON

nutrition info

CALORIES: 262
FAT: 13
CARBS: 30
NET CARBS: 26
FIBER: 4
PROTEIN: 5

MUFFINS

- 3 medium (240 g) carrots, peeled and shredded
- 1 cup (225 g) dried dates, pitted
- ½ cup (56 g) walnuts
- ¼ cup (60 ml) avocado oil
- 2 large eggs, beaten
- ¼ cup (60 g) honey or maple syrup
- 1 teaspoon (5 ml) pure vanilla extract
- 1 tablespoon (6 g) peeled and grated fresh ginger
- ¾ cup (90 g) spelt four
- ¼ cup (34 g) ground flaxseed
- ¾ cup (90 g) almond flour
- ½ teaspoon (3 g) sea salt
- 2 teaspoons (6 g) ground cinnamon
- 2 teaspoons (8 g) baking powder

Preheat the oven to 375°F (190°C) and line a 12-cup muffin tin with paper or silicone liners.

To make the muffins, add the shredded carrots to a large mixing bowl. Pulse the dates and walnuts in a food processor until finely chopped. Add the dates and walnuts to the carrots. Gently fold in the oil, eggs, honey, vanilla, and ginger.

Mix the spelt flour, flaxseed, almond flour, salt, cinnamon, and baking powder in a separate bowl. Fold into the wet ingredients until well combined.

Spoon the batter into the muffin liners until three-quarters full. Bake in the oven for 20 to 25 minutes, or until a toothpick inserted in the center of a muffin comes out clean.

Remove from the oven and transfer to a cooling rack to cool for a few minutes before serving. Store any leftovers in an airtight container for up to 5 days.

curry roasted almonds, cashews, and walnuts

SERVINGS: 12
PREP TIME: 5 MIN
COOK TIME: 30 MIN

DAIRY-FREE
GLUTEN-FREE
VEGAN
VEGETARIAN
GRAIN-FREE

superfoods used

AVOCADO OIL
ALMOND
CASHEW
WALNUT
SESAME SEED
TURMERIC

nutrition info

CALORIES: 223
FAT: 20
CARBS: 10
NET CARBS: 7
FIBER: 3
PROTEIN: 6

A handful of these spiced nuts are a delicious and satisfying snack. Nuts are the fruit of the plant, and we gain substantial benefits when we consume them. Whichever nuts you choose to eat, you are getting anti-inflammatory and antioxidant benefits and a great source of fatty acids. In addition, nuts are a great source of protein that's tasty yet satisfying. You can use any combination of raw nuts that you like. Experiment using pecans, hazelnuts, or chopped Brazil nuts!

SPICED NUTS

- 2 tablespoons (30 ml) avocado oil
- 2 tablespoons (30 g) honey or maple syrup
- 1½ teaspoons (9 g) sea salt
- ½ teaspoon (3 g) black pepper
- 1 tablespoon (7 g) yellow curry powder
- 2 teaspoons (6 g) ground cinnamon
- Sprinkle of dried red pepper flakes
- 1 cup (143 g) raw almonds
- 1 cup (140 g) raw cashews
- 1 cup (120 g) raw walnuts
- ½ cup (35 g) shredded unsweetened coconut
- 1 tablespoon (9 g) black or white sesame seeds

Preheat the oven to 325°F (165°C). Line a baking sheet with parchment paper.

Add all the ingredients to a large mixing bowl. Toss together until everything is evenly coated.

Spread in an even layer on the prepared baking sheet. Bake in the oven for 20 minutes, tossing at the halfway mark. Continue baking for 5 to 10 minutes, or until the nuts are golden in color.

Remove from the oven and transfer the parchment paper and nuts to a cooling rack and completely cool before serving.

Store any leftovers in an airtight container for up to 7 days.

green tea rice bowls with miso-glazed salmon

SERVINGS: 6
PREP TIME: 10 MIN
COOK TIME: 45 MIN

DAIRY-FREE
GLUTEN-FREE
(VEGAN OPTION)

Green tea served over rice is a Japanese tradition (called *ochazuke*). Green tea is high in flavonoids and improves gut health, but also possesses excellent immunoregulating properties. Its earthy flavor is deliciously paired with sweet miso, coconut aminos, and salty salmon in this recipe. Miso is made from fermented soybeans and is rich in minerals and probiotics for gut health.

superfoods used

SESAME SEED
GREEN TEA
SALMON
MISO

RICE

- 1 cup (200 g) brown rice
- 5 cups (1200 ml) water, divided
- 1 tablespoon (15 ml) rice vinegar
- 1 tablespoon (10 g) black or white sesame seeds
- 1 whole (15 g) scallion, minced
- 6 heaping teaspoons (6 g) loose-leaf green tea

SALMON

- 1 tablespoon (17 g) light miso paste
- 2 tablespoons (30 ml) coconut aminos
- 1 teaspoon (6 g) sea salt
- ½ teaspoon (3 g) black pepper
- 10 ounces (285 g) wild-caught, skin-on salmon fillets (or 14 ounces [400 g] extra-firm tofu)

GARNISH

- 1 tablespoon (10 g) black or white sesame seeds
- ½ medium (8 g) scallion, minced

To make the rice, rinse the rice very well using a fine-mesh strainer. Add it with 2 cups (480 ml) of the water to a pot on the stove. Cover and bring to a boil. Once boiling, decrease to a simmer and cook until soft and fluffy, 40 to 45 minutes. Remove from the heat and stir in the rice vinegar, sesame seeds, and scallion. Divide among 6 bowls

To prepare the green tea, place the tea in a teapot or bowl. Heat the remaining 3 cups (720 ml) water to 180°F (82°C) and pour over the tea. Steep for 2 to 3 minutes, then strain the leaves. Pour ½ cup (120 ml) of the green tea on top of the rice in each bowl.

While the rice is cooking, prepare the salmon (or tofu). Preheat the broiler. Line a baking sheet with parchment paper. Mix the miso paste, coconut aminos, salt, and pepper in a small bowl. Pat the salmon (or tofu) dry and place it skin-side down on the prepared baking sheet. Rub it with the miso mixture and broil for 2 minutes. Remove from the oven.

Serve 2 ounces (57 g) of salmon (or tofu) in each bowl of rice, garnishing with the sesame seeds and scallion. Store any leftovers in an airtight container for up to 2 days.

nutrition info

CALORIES: 255
FAT: 8
CARBS: 28
NET CARBS: 26
FIBER: 2
PROTEIN: 13

nutrition info for vegan option

CALORIES: 236
FAT: 6
CARBS: 29
NET CARBS: 27
FIBER: 2
PROTEIN: 13

powerful immunity soup

Astragalus root is known to improve immunity and prevent respiratory infections, such as colds and flus. Its dried root is often sold as a tea, but you can find it as a powder, capsule, or tincture at many health food markets. This recipe combines it all! The variety of vegetables mixed with herbs really gives this recipe a powerful boost. As the ingredients simmer together they release their synergistic immune-boosting properties. This is a go-to recipe when you are feeling under the weather to support your immune system and help you bounce back!

SERVINGS: 8
PREP TIME: 10 MIN
COOK TIME: 30 MIN

VEGETARIAN
VEGAN
DAIRY-FREE
GLUTEN-FREE
GRAIN-FREE

superfoods used

AVOCADO OIL
ONION
GARLIC
ROSEMARY
CARROT
BROCCOLI
ASTRAGALUS
LEMON

nutrition info

CALORIES: 83
FAT: 4
CARBS: 9
NET CARBS: 6
FIBER: 3
PROTEIN: 3

SOUP

- 2 tablespoons (30 ml) avocado oil
- 1 medium (150 g) yellow onion, chopped
- 4 small (16 g) cloves garlic, minced
- 1 teaspoon (6 g) sea salt
- ½ teaspoon (3 g) black pepper
- 1 tablespoon (3 g) dried rosemary
- 1 cup (150 g) chopped carrots
- 4 cups (360 g) chopped cremini mushrooms
- 2 cups (142 g) broccoli florets
- ¼ cup (12 g) dried astragalus root
- 4 cups (960 ml) vegetable stock
- 2 tablespoons (30 ml) fresh lemon juice
- 1 tablespoon (15 ml) coconut aminos
- 2 bay leaves
- ¼ cup (4 g) fresh parsley, minced
- ¼ cup (4 g) fresh cilantro, minced
- 1 medium (15 g) scallion, minced

To make the soup, heat the oil in a large pot over medium-low heat. Add the onion, garlic, salt, pepper, and rosemary. Sauté until it begins to soften, about 5 minutes. Add the carrots and continue to sauté for 3 minutes. Add the mushrooms, broccoli, and astragalus and sauté for 3 minutes.

Add the vegetable stock, lemon juice, coconut aminos, and bay leaves. Reduce the heat to low and simmer, uncovered, for 10 minutes. Discard the bay leaves. Stir in the parsley, cilantro, and scallion.

Serve and enjoy! Store any leftovers in the fridge in an airtight container for up to 5 days.

southwestern quinoa salad

with yellow squash and black beans

SERVINGS: 8
PREP TIME: 10 MIN
PLUS SOAKING
OVERNIGHT
COOK TIME: 35 MIN

This salad has yellow squash, less popular than green, but a wonderful choice, as it is high in potassium and magnesium. Pumpkin seeds are an excellent source of iron, magnesium, and zinc—all of which are critical to immune health. Pumpkin seeds also are gaining popularity because they are an excellent protein source. Serve this salad on its own, or try it in a gluten-free tortilla, with scrambled eggs, or as a salad with chicken!

VEGAN
VEGETARIAN
DAIRY-FREE
GLUTEN-FREE

QUINOA

- 1 cup (200 g) quinoa (soaked overnight in cold water)
- 1¼ cups (300 ml) boiling water

SALAD

- ¼ cup (60 ml) olive oil
- 2 tablespoons (30 ml) fresh lime juice
- ¼ cup (4 g) fresh cilantro, minced
- 1 teaspoon (6 g) sea salt
- ½ teaspoon (3 g) black pepper
- 1 teaspoon (4 g) smoked paprika
- 1 teaspoon (5) ground cumin
- 1 teaspoon (2 g) chili powder
- 1 medium (200 g) yellow squash, shredded
- 1 medium (150 g) yellow, orange, or red bell pepper, seeded and diced
- 1 medium (40 g) shallot, minced
- 15 ounces (425 g) cooked black beans, rinsed
- ¼ cup (28 g) raw pepitas

To prepare the quinoa, rinse the soaked quinoa very well using a fine-mesh strainer, then transfer to a saucepan and add the boiling water over low heat. Let the quinoa soak in the boiling water for about 10 minutes, or until it has soaked up all the water.

To make the salad, add the olive oil to a large mixing bowl, followed by the lime juice, cilantro, salt, pepper, smoked paprika, cumin, and chili powder.

Add the yellow squash, bell pepper, shallot, black beans, and pepitas to the bowl and gently toss in the mixture until everything is coated. Add the cooked quinoa, and gently toss until fully coated.

Serve and enjoy! Store any leftovers in the fridge in an airtight container for up to 5 days.

superfoods used

QUINOA
OLIVE OIL
LIME
YELLOW SQUASH
BELL PEPPER
PUMPKIN SEEDS

nutrition info

CALORIES: 260
FAT: 10
CARBS: 33
NET CARBS: 25
FIBER: 8
PROTEIN: 10

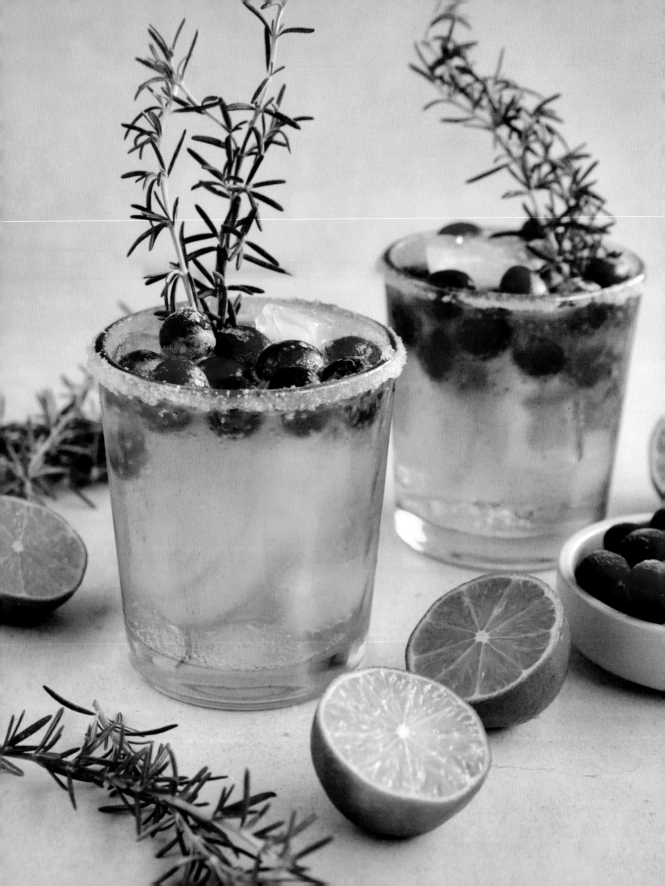

CHAPTER SIX

DRINKS & ELIXIRS

When we talk about herbs, most people associate them with a cup of hot tea to soothe them when they are not feeling well. Herbs do have valuable healing properties—but you also can incorporate many herbs as a preventative to keep you healthy and thriving! In this chapter, you'll learn how to combine herbs that support your immune system in refreshing elixirs you can make right at home.

Many of you already may be familiar with golden milk latte. Well, here you will find the Twice Golden Milk Latte (page 77)! It uses goldenseal to give a boost of gut-healing properties to this enjoyable drink. Or try the Soothing Licorice-Lavender Latte (page 78) to calm the nervous system. Lavender has been shown to be as effective as prescription benzodiazepines to reduce anxiety. The addition of licorice gives it just the right amount of sweetness, and it also helps with leaky gut.

This is just the beginning to get you thinking about how to incorporate herbs into your daily life. It's yet another simple way to get to the goal of consuming nine to twelve servings of plants each and every day. These herbs count toward that goal and are loaded with anti-inflammatory, antioxidant, and immune-boosting properties.

Sparkling Cranberry-Lime
Mocktail, page 85

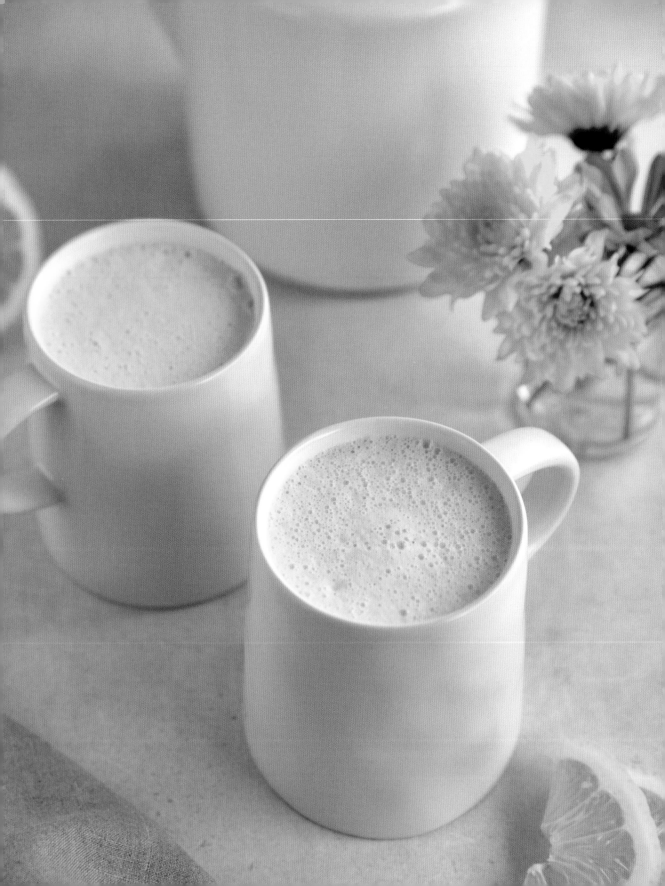

twice golden milk latte

Here is a little twist on the ever so popular golden milk, with the added touch of goldenseal! Goldenseal root is known to reduce inflammation and boost immunity. It contains berberine, which has been shown to improve gut dysbiosis and improve small intestinal bacterial overgrowth. Turmeric adds to this anti-inflammatory mechanism with its ability to block the king of inflammation, NF-kB. Add in the antioxidant benefits of cloves and glucose-regulating ability of cinnamon and you have the perfect immune, gut, and antioxidant super drink! Note: Due to its powerful nature, goldenseal is not recommended for those pregnant or breastfeeding.

SERVINGS: 2
PREP TIME: 5 MIN
COOK TIME: 15 MIN

VEGAN
VEGETARIAN
DAIRY-FREE
GLUTEN-FREE
GRAIN-FREE

superfoods used

GOLDENSEAL
TURMERIC
CINNAMON
CLOVES
LEMON

nutrition info

CALORIES: 239
FAT: 13
CARBS: 31
NET CARBS: 28
FIBER: 3
PROTEIN: 2

LATTE

- 2 cups (480 ml) almond milk or your choice of plant-based milk
- 2 bags (2.6 g) goldenseal tea
- 1 teaspoon (5 g) ground turmeric
- ¼ teaspoon (0.75 g) ground cinnamon
- Pinch of ground cloves
- Pinch of ground nutmeg
- Pinch of sea salt
- Pinch of black pepper
- 2 tablespoons (30 g) coconut butter
- 1 teaspoon (5 ml) fresh lemon juice
- 1 tablespoon (15 ml) honey or maple syrup

To make the latte, add the almond milk to a small saucepot over medium-low heat. When it begins to boil, turn off the heat and add the goldenseal. Let sit for 10 minutes, then strain through a fine-mesh sieve, returning the almond milk to the pot.

Add the remaining ingredients and bring to a simmer. Once simmering, turn off the heat and serve warm.

soothing licorice-lavender latte

SERVINGS: 2
PREP TIME: 5 MIN
COOK TIME: 15 MIN

VEGETARIAN
VEGAN
DAIRY-FREE
GLUTEN-FREE
GRAIN-FREE

superfoods used

LICORICE

nutrition info

CALORIES: 173
FAT: 11
CARBS: 17
NET CARBS: 14
FIBER: 3
PROTEIN: 2

Lavender is calming, making this latte a wonderful evening beverage. Opt for English culinary varieties, as French lavender is better suited for bath and body use. Licorice soothes inflammation and improves digestion, a great herbal remedy to improve leaky gut. The coconut butter adds richness to this drink. Simply sweeten it with honey for the perfect blend. It's important to look for local, pure, unprocessed honey to gain excellent anti-allergy benefits. Note: Due to its powerful nature, licorice is not recommended for those pregnant or breastfeeding.

LATTE

- 2 cups (480 ml) water
- 2 bags (2 g) licorice root tea
- ½ teaspoon (1 g) dried English lavender buds
- 1 cup (240 ml) almond milk or your choice of plant-based milk
- ¼ teaspoon (1 g) pure vanilla bean powder
- Pinch of sea salt
- 2 tablespoons (30 g) coconut butter
- 1 tablespoon (15 ml) honey or maple syrup

To make the latte, bring the water to a boil (200°F [93°C]) in a kettle and turn off the heat. Pour the water over the tea bags and dried lavender in a heatproof bowl. Let steep for 10 minutes. When done, discard the tea bags and strain through a fine-mesh sieve.

Add the tea to a small saucepot, followed by the remaining ingredients, stirring well. Bring to a simmer, then turn off the heat. Serve and enjoy!

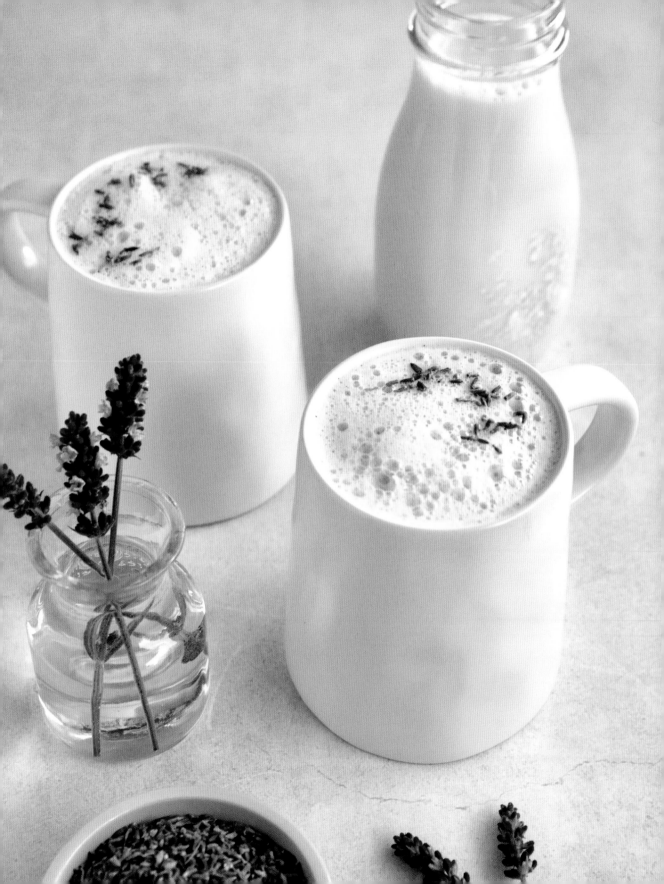

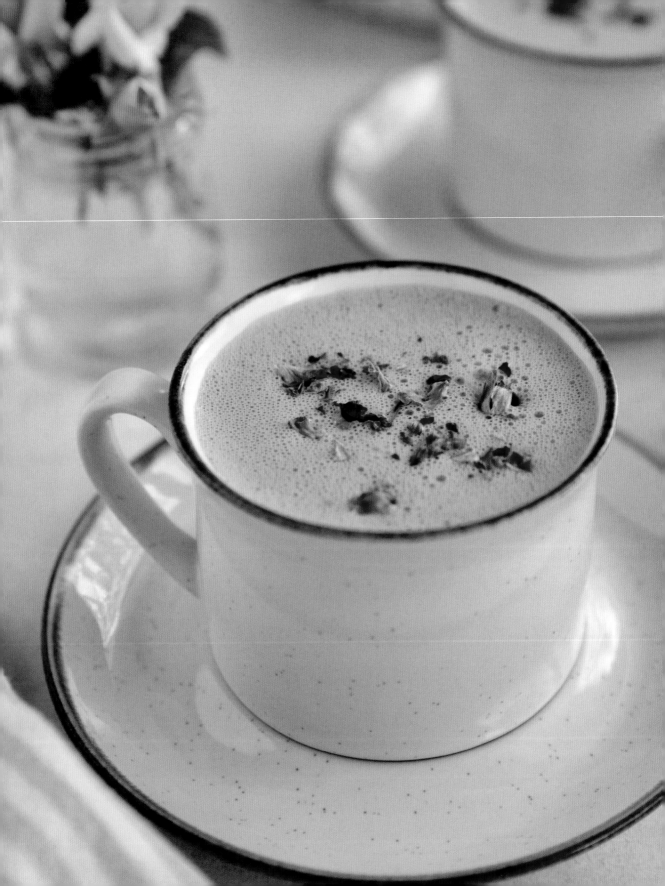

chocolate rose latte

Chocolate and rose make such a delicious pairing. Cacao is packed with phenolics, primarily flavonoids, that give it its high antioxidant capacity and strong anti-inflammatory potential. We boost the anti-inflammatory properties with the addition of andrographis. Andrographis blocks the release of pro-inflammatory cytokines as a result of its anti-inflammatory mechanism. It is known to be immune-stimulating, so keep that in mind if you already have an upregulated immune system due to autoimmunity. Sip it to unwind after a full day and pause to reap its calming benefits.

SERVINGS: 2
PREP TIME: 5 MIN
COOK TIME: 15 MIN

VEGETARIAN
VEGAN
DAIRY-FREE
GLUTEN-FREE
GRAIN-FREE

superfoods used

ANDROGRAPHIS

nutrition info

CALORIES: 189
FAT: 12
CARBS: 17
NET CARBS: 12
FIBER: 5
PROTEIN: 3

LATTE

- 2 cups (480 ml) water
- 2 bags (2 g) rose tea
- 1 cup (240 ml) almond milk or your choice of plant-based milk
- 2 tablespoons (15 g) cacao powder
- ¼ teaspoon (1 g) pure vanilla bean powder
- Pinch of sea salt
- ⅛ teaspoon ground cardamom
- 2 tablespoons (30 g) coconut butter
- 2 tablespoons (30 ml) maple syrup
- 1 serving andrographis tincture

GARNISH

- 1 teaspoon (1 g) dried culinary-grade rosebuds

To make the latte, bring the water to a boil (200°F [93°C]) in a kettle and turn off the heat. Pour the water over the tea bags in a heatproof bowl. Let steep for 10 minutes. When done, discard the tea bags.

Add the tea to a small saucepot, followed by the remaining ingredients, stirring well. Bring to a simmer, then turn off the heat. Serve garnished with dried rosebuds.

sunset fruit punch

VEGETARIAN
VEGAN
DAIRY-FREE
GLUTEN-FREE
GRAIN-FREE

superfoods used

APPLE
ORANGE
CRANBERRY

nutrition info

CALORIES: 115
FAT: 0
CARBS: 29
NET CARBS: 29
FIBER: 0
PROTEIN: 1

The glow of this punch will remind you of the antioxidants found in apples, oranges, and cranberries. Antioxidants are essential to protect our cells from damage by reactive oxygen species in the body. This combination is also the ultimate vitamin C boost; all three of these fruits are packed with immune-boosting vitamin C. Serve this at a social gathering, or better yet, as a healthy clean juice for kids. Enjoy the sweetness of nature!

PUNCH

- 4 cups (800 g) ice cubes
- 32 ounces (912 ml) fresh apple juice
- 32 ounces (912 ml) fresh orange juice
- 32 ounces (912 ml) fresh cranberry juice
- 32 ounces (912 ml) plain or lemon seltzer

GARNISH

Fresh orange slices

Fresh mint

To make the punch, add the ice cubes to a punch bowl. Add all of the juices and the seltzer, and stir to combine. Serve garnished with fresh orange slices and mint.

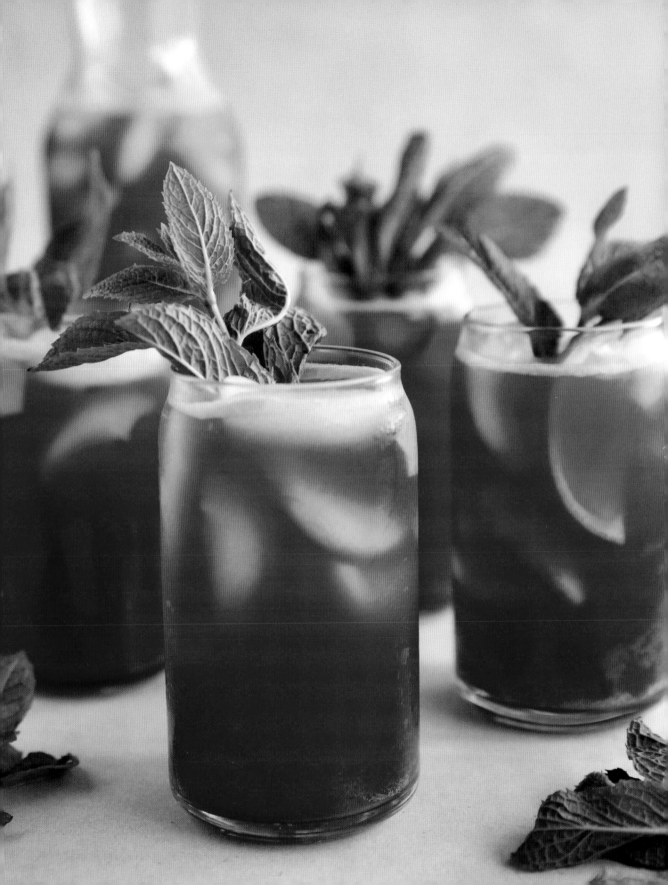

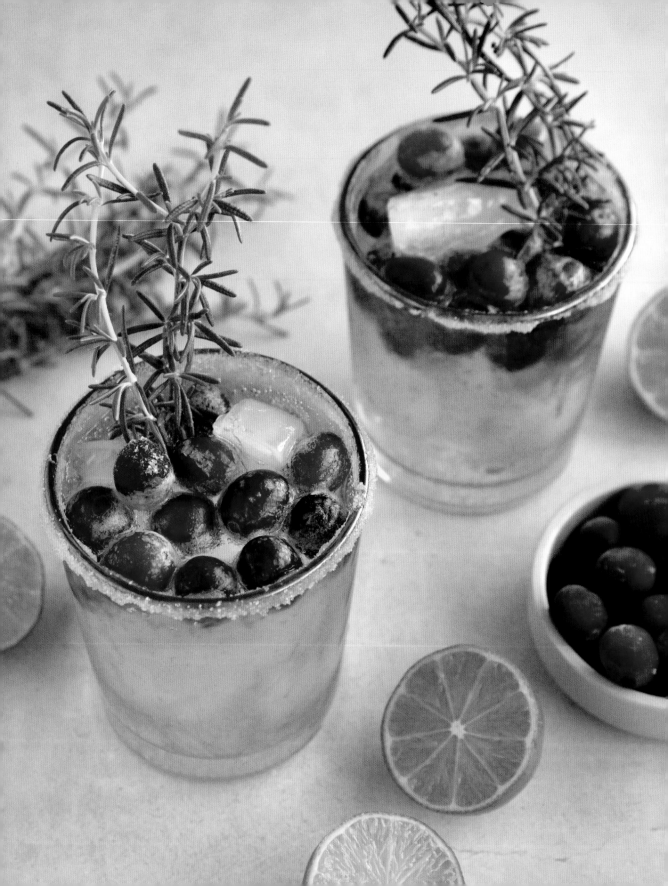

sparkling cranberry-lime mocktail

Cranberries are rich in antioxidants, so aim to include them in your recipes. They often are sold fresh during the holiday season, but they can be found year-round in the freezer section of your market. If using dried cranberries, opt for apple juice–sweetened varieties in sunflower oil instead of traditional sugar and canola oil. The addition of lime in this recipe can't go unnoticed. Limes contain antioxidants, which help to reduce inflammation. Limes, like many other citrus varieties, are very high in vitamin C, which is essential for our immune system.

MOCKTAIL

- ½ cup (120 ml) water
- 2 tablespoons (30 g) coconut sugar (optional)
- 8–10 ice cubes
- 2 bottles (24 ounces, or 684 ml) lime seltzer
- 2 tablespoons (30 ml) fresh lime juice
- ½ cup (100 g) fresh or frozen cranberries
- 2 sprigs fresh rosemary

To make the mocktail, place two small bowls on the counter. Add the water to one and the coconut sugar, if using, to the other. Dip the top ½ inch (1 cm) of two glasses in the water, then in the coconut sugar, lining the rims. Set upright on the counter.

Fill each glass with 4 or 5 ice cubes, then add the lime seltzer, lime juice, cranberries, and sprigs of rosemary. Serve and enjoy!

SERVINGS: 2
PREP TIME: 5 MIN
COOK TIME: 0 MIN

VEGETARIAN
VEGAN
DAIRY-FREE
GLUTEN-FREE
GRAIN-FREE

superfoods used

CRANBERRIES
LIME
ROSEMARY

nutrition info

CALORIES: 82
FAT: 0
CARBS: 19
NET CARBS: 13
FIBER: 6
PROTEIN: 1

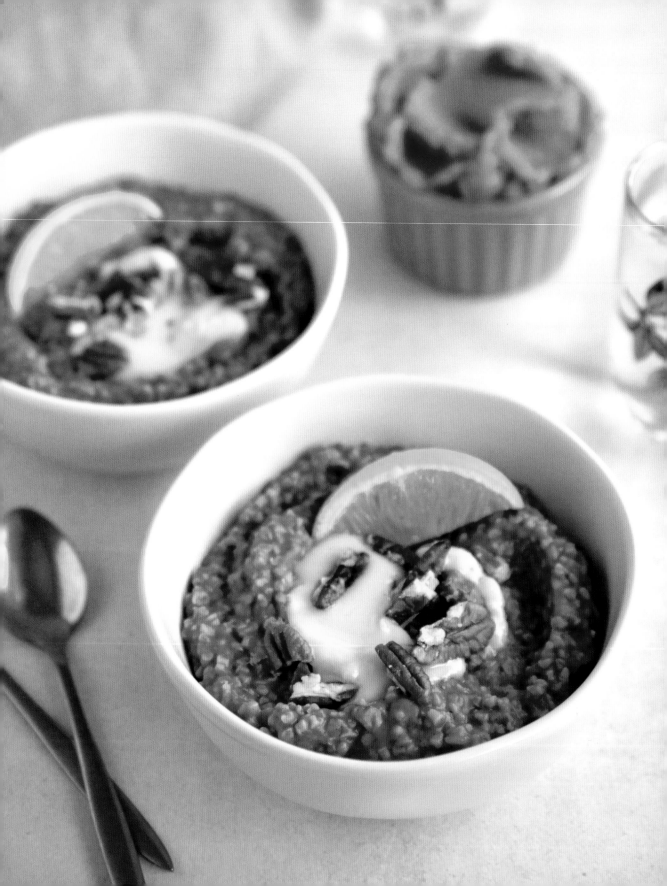

CHAPTER SEVEN

BREAKFAST & BRUNCH

Some say breakfast is the most important meal of the day, but quite frankly I think all meals are important! Ensuring we are not skipping breakfast, which many of us do, is what's most important to guarantee we are hitting a target of plant-based foods we feed our body each and every day. In my experience, I have found many people just get bored with breakfast, and if you're like me and can't consume eggs, then you are forced to get creative. That is exactly what you will find in these recipes—variety. These recipes are satisfying and tasty and not just another omelet, although there are plenty of egg options!

You can spice up that plain oatmeal with pumpkin and cardamom for a fun fall breakfast. Many don't think of quinoa as a breakfast option, but why not? As a great source of protein in the morning, it helps keep you full longer and is packed with nutrients. You will love the Sprouted Quinoa Porridge with Raspberries and Hazelnut Butter (page 89). If smoothies are your thing, don't worry, I have plenty of options that are nutrient dense and taste great too. One recipe you have to try is the Grounding Daily Kichadi (page 109). This is an ancient Indian dish that is packed with immune-boosting foods, herbs, and spices. You can pair it with eggs, or even one of the beverages from chapter 6! Go on, get creative with your breakfast and make it the most exciting meal of the day!

Pumpkin Cardamom Oats
with Coconut Butter and Orange
Zest, page 90

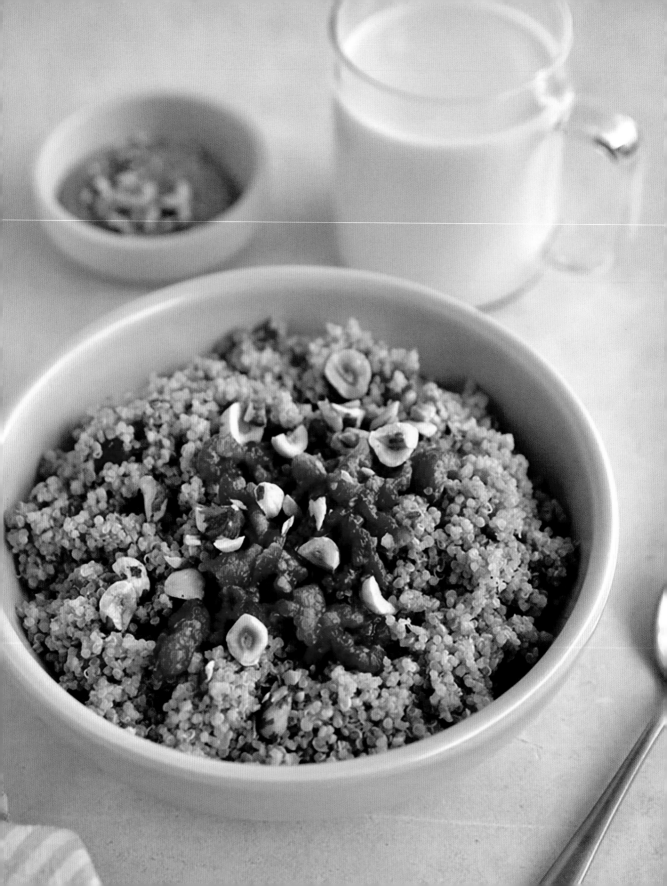

sprouted quinoa porridge with raspberries and hazelnut butter

SERVINGS: 2
PREP TIME: 10 MIN
PLUS SOAKING
OVERNIGHT
COOK TIME: 15 MIN

VEGETARIAN
VEGAN
DAIRY-FREE
GLUTEN-FREE

superfoods used

QUINOA
RASPBERRY
HAZELNUT

Grown primarily for its edible seeds, quinoa is an excellent source of plant-based protein. It is rich in fiber, B vitamins, and minerals such as magnesium. It's also loaded with fiber, a great way to start the morning. The raspberries in this recipe are high in fiber as well, helping you hit that daily goal of 30 grams. They are also excellent for your gut. Raspberries help balance good and bad bacteria in the gut, thereby reducing inflammation. Nuts give you that added anti-inflammatory benefit and good fat, keeping you full longer. Use this porridge recipe as a base and swap the raspberries and hazelnuts for other fruits and nuts, such as blueberries and walnuts, or cherries and almonds.

PORRIDGE

- 1 cup (200 g) quinoa (soaked overnight in cold water)
- 1¼ cups (300 ml) boiling water
- 1 cup (240 ml) plain, unsweetened hazelnut milk or your choice of plant-based milk

  Pinch of sea salt

- ¼ cup (31 g) fresh raspberries
- 1 tablespoon (16 g) hazelnut butter

GARNISH

- ¼ cup (31 g) fresh raspberries
- 2 tablespoons (14 g) chopped hazelnuts

To make the porridge, rinse the soaked quinoa very well using a fine-mesh strainer, then transfer to a saucepot over low heat and add the boiling water. Let the quinoa soak in the boiling water for about 10 minutes, or until it has soaked up all the water.

Add the hazelnut milk and simmer for about 5 minutes, stirring often to prevent the quinoa from sticking. Stir in the salt, raspberries, and hazelnut butter until thoroughly combined.

Serve garnished with the raspberries and chopped hazelnuts. Store any leftovers in the fridge in an airtight container for up to 3 days.

nutrition info

CALORIES: 541
FAT: 18
CARBS: 74
NET CARBS: 64
FIBER: 10
PROTEIN: 18

pumpkin cardamom oats

with coconut butter and orange zest

SERVINGS: 2
PREP TIME: 5 MIN
COOK TIME: 10 MIN

VEGETARIAN
VEGAN
DAIRY-FREE
GLUTEN-FREE

superfoods used

CINNAMON
PECAN
ORANGE

nutrition info

CALORIES: 377
FAT: 21
CARBS: 38
NET CARBS: 31
FIBER: 7
PROTEIN: 8

The autumn season is when we see pumpkin recipes at their peak, but you can prepare this dish anytime by using canned pumpkin puree. Just be sure to choose brands using only pumpkin in the ingredients. Oatmeal is an excellent option for breakfast for multiple reasons: It contains avenanthramides, antioxidants that are solely found in oats, which help lower blood pressure by increasing the production of nitric oxide. Oats are also high in beta-glucan, a type of soluble fiber that promotes the release of peptide YY, a satiety hormone produced in the gut that increases the feeling of fullness.

PUMPKIN CARDAMOM OATS

- 1½ cups (360 ml) plain, unsweetened almond milk or your choice of plant-based milk
- 1 cup (120 g) raw steel-cut oats
- ½ cup (113 g) pumpkin puree
- Pinch of sea salt
- 1 teaspoon (3 g) pumpkin pie spice
- ½ teaspoon (2 g) ground cinnamon
- ¼ teaspoon (1 g) ground cardamom

GARNISH

- 2 tablespoons (31 g) coconut butter, melted
- 2 tablespoons (16 g) chopped pecans
- Zest from ½ medium (15 g) fresh orange

To make the oats, add the almond milk, oats, pumpkin puree, salt, pumpkin pie spice, cinnamon, and cardamom to a saucepot. Bring to a boil. Once boiling, reduce the heat to a simmer and stir often for about 5 minutes.

Remove from the heat and serve with the melted coconut butter, pecans, and orange zest. Store any leftovers in the fridge in an airtight container for up to 3 days.

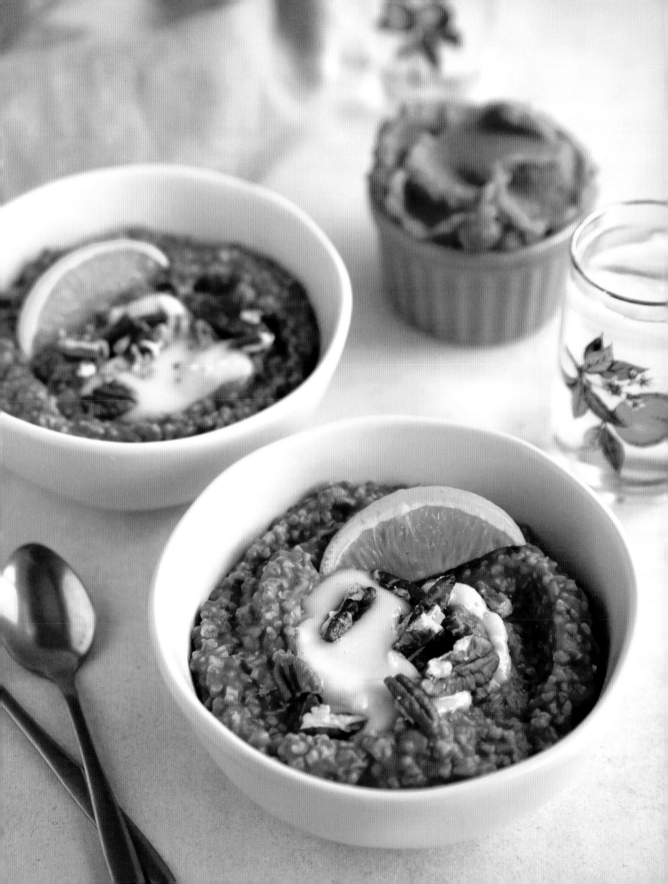

beet-and-orange spice smoothie

SERVINGS: 2
PREP TIME: 5 MIN
COOK TIME: 0 MIN

VEGETARIAN
VEGAN
DAIRY-FREE
GLUTEN-FREE
GRAIN-FREE

superfoods used

BEET
ORANGE
BANANA
ALMOND
CINNAMON
CLOVE

nutrition info

CALORIES: 304
FAT: 11
CARBS: 49
NET CARBS: 36
FIBER: 13
PROTEIN: 8

Beets make an unexpected and delicious addition to a smoothie. Did you know beets can be useful in preventing fatty liver disease? They contain a nutritious substance called betaine, which is made in the liver and reduces hepatic enzymes, steatosis, and fibrosis in NASH patients. Betalains have a high antioxidant potential and anti-inflammatory properties. Beetroot is a natural nitric oxide donor, which has a positive effect on our blood vessels. You can add extra fat or protein to this smoothie with chia seeds, a handful of chickpeas, or a sprinkle of pistachios.

SMOOTHIE

- 2 cups (480 ml) plain, unsweetened almond milk or your choice of plant-based milk
- 1½ cups (200 g) peeled and chopped beets
- 1 cup (300 g) fresh orange segments
- 1 cup (150 g) sliced frozen banana
- 2 tablespoons (32 g) raw almond butter or nut butter of choice
- 1 teaspoon (3 g) ground cinnamon
- ½ teaspoon (1.5) ground cardamom
- ⅛ teaspoon ground nutmeg
- Pinch of ground cloves
- Pinch of black pepper
- Pinch of sea salt

To make the smoothie, add all the ingredients to a blender. Blend on high speed until very creamy. Serve immediately.

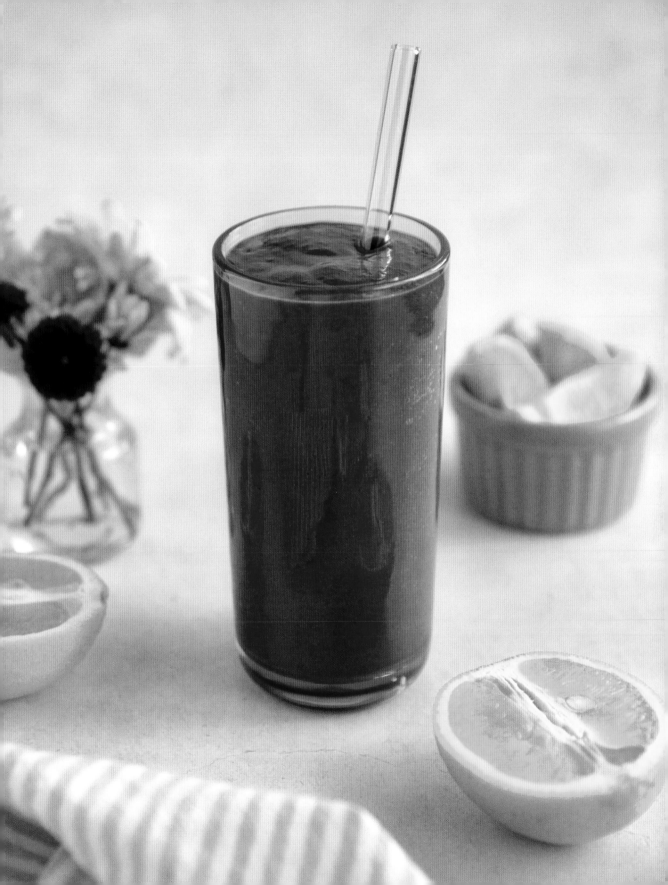

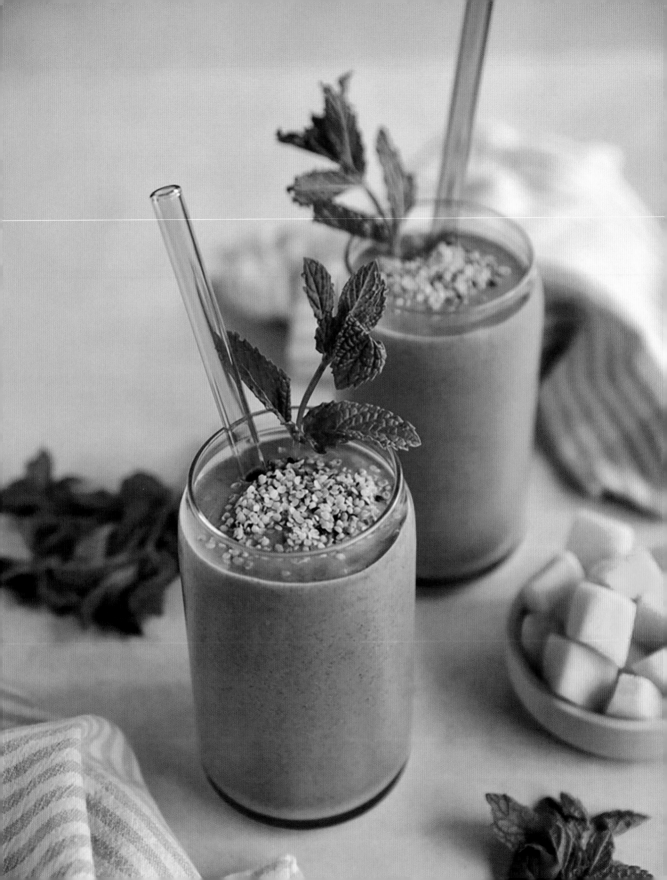

minty mango green smoothie

This smoothie is rich in vitamins and minerals, making it an excellent way to start your day. Cinnamon, cloves, and fresh peppermint create a unique and surprisingly delicious combination! Chia seeds are a great source of PUFAs (good fats), and are also rich in fiber and antioxidants. You definitely can't go wrong. The mango gives you all the benefits of mangiferin, a potent antioxidant and anti-inflammatory that stimulates SCFA production and is excellent for our gut bacteria.

SERVINGS: 2
PREP TIME: 5 MIN
COOK TIME: 0 MIN

VEGETARIAN
VEGAN
DAIRY-FREE
GLUTEN-FREE
GRAIN-FREE

superfoods used

MANGO
BANANA
CHIA SEED
PEPPERMINT
CINNAMON
HEMP SEED
CLOVES

nutrition info

CALORIES: 367
FAT: 15
CARBS: 47
NET CARBS: 32
FIBER: 15
PROTEIN: 14

SMOOTHIE

- 2 cups (480 ml) plain, unsweetened almond milk or your choice of plant-based milk
- 1¼ cups (140 g) fresh or frozen mango chunks
- 4 cups (200 g) baby spinach
- 1 medium (115 g) frozen banana
- 3 tablespoons (39 g) chia seeds
- 4 fresh peppermint leaves
- 1 teaspoon (3 g) ground cinnamon
- Pinch of ground cloves
- Pinch of sea salt

GARNISH

- 3 tablespoons (30 g) hemp seeds
- 2–4 fresh peppermint leaves

To make the smoothie, add all the ingredients to a blender. Blend on high speed until very creamy and green in color. Garnish with the hemp seeds and peppermint leaves. Serve immediately.

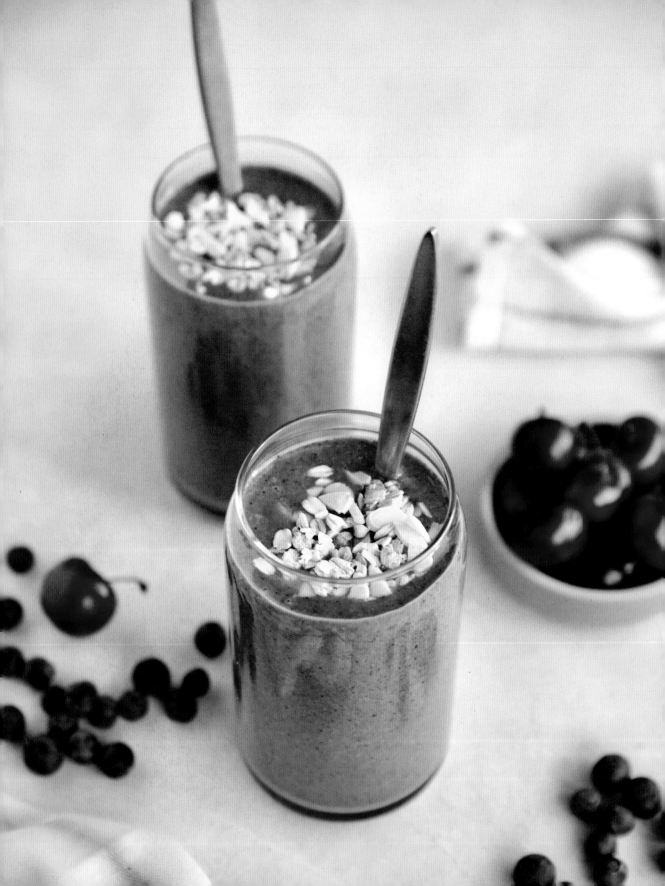

banana-blueberry-cherry smoothie

The addition of oats in this smoothie gives it amazing texture. Oats also contain fiber, which helps improve blood sugar regulation. Blueberries are excellent in smoothies because of their high fiber content, which is essential for our gut and keeps us full longer. Cherries also are a bonus for the gut, as they help increase Bifidobacterium in the gut. (This bacteria plays an important role in balancing our immune system.)

SERVINGS: 2
PREP TIME: 5 MIN
COOK TIME: 0 MIN

VEGETARIAN
VEGAN
DAIRY-FREE
GLUTEN-FREE

SMOOTHIE

- 2 cups (480 ml) plain, unsweetened almond milk or your choice of plant-based milk
- 1 medium (115 g) sliced frozen banana
- 1 cup (100 g) frozen and pitted cherries
- ½ cup (48 g) blueberries
- ½ cup (45 g) dry sprouted oats
- 2 tablespoons (32 g) raw almond butter or nut butter of choice
- 1 teaspoon (3 g) ground cinnamon
- 2 tablespoons (26 g) chia seeds
- Pinch of sea salt

To make the smoothie, add all the ingredients to a blender. Blend on high speed until very creamy. Serve immediately.

superfoods used

BANANA
BLUEBERRY
ALMOND
CINNAMON
CHIA SEED
CHERRY

nutrition info

CALORIES: 406
FAT: 15
CARBS: 60
NET CARBS: 45
FIBER: 15
PROTEIN: 11

chamomile spelt porridge

with cinnamon apples

SERVINGS: 4
PREP TIME: 10 MIN
COOK TIME: 20 MIN

VEGETARIAN
VEGAN
DAIRY-FREE
GLUTEN-FREE

superfoods used

SPELT
CHAMOMILE
APPLE
CINNAMON
WALNUT
AVOCADO OIL

nutrition info

CALORIES: 215
FAT: 7
CARBS: 34
NET CARBS: 28
FIBER: 6
PROTEIN: 5

Chamomile is so flavorful on its own, but imagine what it can do to your plain grains. It is also incredibly gut healing, a great way to start the day. Spelt is an ancient grain packed with protein; although not gluten-free, it is much easier to digest. You can crack your own whole spelt by placing it in a food processor and pulsing until it is broken up. The benefit of cracking your spelt before cooking is much less time exposed to oxygen, which increases oxidation when the spelt is split open and no longer in its whole form. It is an extra step in this recipe, but worth it!

CHAMOMILE SPELT PORRIDGE

- 2 bags chamomile tea
- 2 cups (480 ml) boiling water
- 1 cup (120 g) cracked spelt
- 1 cup (240 ml) plain, unsweetened almond milk or your choice of plant-based milk
- Pinch of sea salt

CINNAMON APPLES

- 1 tablespoon (15 g) avocado oil
- 2 medium (230 g) apples, cored and chopped
- Pinch of sea salt
- 1 tablespoon (8 g) ground cinnamon

GARNISH

- ½ of the cinnamon apple recipe
- ¼ cup (28 g) chopped walnuts

To make the porridge, in a heatproof bowl, steep the tea bags in the boiling water for 5 minutes. Discard the tea bags. Add the chamomile tea, cracked spelt, and almond milk to a saucepot. Bring to a boil, then decrease to a simmer and cook until the spelt is tender, about 20 minutes.

While the spelt is simmering, prepare your cinnamon apples. Warm the oil in a large skillet over medium-low heat. Add the apples, salt, and cinnamon and toss together until the apples are coated. Sauté over low heat until the apples are soft and fragrant, 5 to 10 minutes. Turn off the heat.

When the spelt is done cooking, turn off the heat and stir in half of the cinnamon apples until well combined. Top your porridge with the remaining cinnamon apples and walnuts.

Serve and enjoy! Store any leftovers in the fridge in an airtight container for up to 7 days.

orange cream smoothie

This smoothie is packed with vitamin C and fiber. Oranges are a no-brainer when it comes to immune-boosting foods. Beyond being famous for vitamin C, they also are known to reduce inflammation due to their flavonoid content. Boost this recipe with the almond butter; it gives you 6 grams of protein and 4 grams of fiber! The added nut butter also provides healthy fats to help you absorb the vitamins and minerals in this recipe, and it adds an amazing flavor and creamy texture!

SERVINGS: 2
PREP TIME: 5 MIN
COOK TIME: 0 MIN

VEGETARIAN
VEGAN
DAIRY-FREE
GLUTEN-FREE
GRAIN-FREE

superfoods used

BANANA
ORANGE
ALMOND
CINNAMON

SMOOTHIE

- 2 cups (480 ml) plain, unsweetened almond milk or your choice of plant-based milk
- 1 cup (235 g) plain coconut yogurt
- 1 cup (150 g) sliced frozen banana
- 1 cup (300 g) fresh orange segments
- 2 tablespoons (32 g) raw almond butter or nut butter of choice
- 1 teaspoon (4 g) vanilla bean powder
- 1 teaspoon (3 g) ground cinnamon
- Pinch of sea salt

To make the smoothie, add all the ingredients to a blender. Blend on high speed until very creamy. Serve immediately.

nutrition info

CALORIES: 377
FAT: 16
CARBS: 53
NET CARBS: 44
FIBER: 9
PROTEIN: 8

overnight persimmon-pecan chia pudding

SERVINGS: 2
PREP TIME: 5 MIN
PLUS TIME FOR CHIA
TO THICKEN
COOK TIME: 0 MIN

VEGETARIAN
VEGAN
DAIRY-FREE
GLUTEN-FREE
GRAIN-FREE

superfoods used

PERSIMMON
CHIA SEED
CINNAMON
PECAN
CLOVE

nutrition info

CALORIES: 366
FAT: 20
CARBS: 39
NET CARBS: 20
FIBER: 19
PROTEIN: 10

Preparing this the night before you plan to serve the pudding is best. Chia seed pudding has grown in popularity, and really you can top it with just about any fruit you enjoy. Persimmon is used in this recipe to keep the variety flowing. Persimmons are an excellent choice, especially when in season. They are jam-packed with polyphenols, which have incredible antioxidant potential. If you don't have much time, you can blend this pudding with a banana to increase its thick texture and chill in the fridge for about 1 hour before serving.

PUDDING

- 2 cups (480 ml) plain, unsweetened almond milk or your choice of plant-based milk
- 5 tablespoons (65 g) chia seeds
- 2 teaspoons (6 g) ground cinnamon
- Pinch of ground cloves
- Pinch of ground cardamom
- Pinch of sea salt

GARNISH

- 1 medium (168 g) fresh persimmon, diced
- ¼ cup (28 g) pecans, chopped

To make the pudding, add the almond milk, chia seeds, cinnamon, cloves, cardamom, and salt to a blender. Blend on high speed until well combined.

Pour into two bowls and cover them, or use mason jars and seal them with a lid. Place in the fridge to thicken the night before you plan to serve.

When ready to eat, garnish with the persimmon and pecans. Store any leftovers in the fridge in an airtight container for up to 5 days.

papaya and coconut yogurt breakfast bowls

SERVINGS: 2
PREP TIME: 10 MIN
COOK TIME: 0 MIN

VEGETARIAN
VEGAN
DAIRY-FREE
GLUTEN-FREE
GRAIN-FREE

There is nothing like fresh papaya, so be sure to pick one up so that you can make this delicious breakfast! Papayas are unique in that they possess enzymes only found in this fruit. These enzymes help you break down food, and they also have gut-healing properties. Another great fruit to give you that boost of fiber you need! A tip for finding the perfect papaya is to smell it. If it smells sweet and slightly musky, it's ready to be sliced open and enjoyed!

BREAKFAST BOWLS

- 1 teaspoon (4 g) vanilla bean powder
- 1 cup (235 g) plain coconut yogurt
- 1 medium (275 g) fresh papaya, halved and seeded

GARNISH

- 2 teaspoons (9 g) chia seeds
- 2 tablespoons (20 g) hemp seeds
- 2 tablespoons (14 g) pepitas
- 2 tablespoons (20 g) dried goji berries
- 2 teaspoons (1 g) fresh mint, minced

To make the bowls, stir the vanilla bean powder into the coconut yogurt. Fill each papaya half with the coconut yogurt.

Garnish each papaya half with the chia seeds, hemp seeds, pepitas, goji berries, and mint.

Serve and enjoy! Store any leftovers in the fridge in an airtight container for up to 3 days.

superfoods used

**PAPAYA
CHIA SEED
HEMP SEED
PUMPKIN SEED
PEPPERMINT**

nutrition info

**CALORIES: 357
FAT: 15
CARBS: 47
NET CARBS: 37
FIBER: 10
PROTEIN: 10**

tempeh and breakfast fajitas in jicama shells

SERVINGS: 4
PREP TIME: 10 MIN
COOK TIME: 20 MIN

VEGAN
VEGETARIAN
DAIRY-FREE
GLUTEN-FREE
(NON-VEGAN OPTION)

superfoods used

AVOCADO OIL
ONION
GARLIC
BELL PEPPER
JICAMA
AVOCADO
TEMPEH

nutrition info

CALORIES: 372
FAT: 15
CARBS: 52
NET CARBS: 41
FIBER: 9
PROTEIN: 23

*nutrition info for
non-vegan option*

CALORIES: 406
FAT: 19
CARBS: 31
NET CARBS: 24
FIBER: 7
PROTEIN: 26

Tempeh, made of fermented soybeans, is a great source of plant-based protein. Fermentation increases its antioxidant potential. You can substitute ground chicken or turkey if you prefer. For even more protein and fiber, serve this with a side of black or pinto beans. Many grocery stores sell sliced jicama taco shells in the produce department with the prepackaged leafy greens and vegetables.

FAJITAS

- 12 ounces (340 g) tempeh, crumbled (or 1 pound [454 g] ground chicken)
- 1 tablespoon (15 ml) avocado oil
- ½ medium (75 g) yellow or red onion, minced
- 3 small (12 g) cloves garlic, minced
- 1 teaspoon (6 g) sea salt
- ½ teaspoon (3 g) black pepper
- 1 teaspoon (5 g) smoked paprika
- 1 teaspoon (5) ground cumin
- 1 teaspoon (5 g) chili powder
- 1 medium (150 g) red bell pepper, seeded and sliced
- 1 medium (150 g) green bell pepper, seeded and sliced
- Zest from ½ medium (11 g) fresh lime
- 1 tablespoon (15 ml) fresh lime juice
- 8 jicama taco shells or 8 (¼ inch, or 6 mm) round slices of fresh jicama

GARNISH

- 1 medium (150 g) avocado, peeled and chopped
- ¼ cup (4 g) fresh cilantro, minced

If preparing the non-vegan option, add the chicken to a large, nonstick skillet over medium-low heat. Sauté until fully cooked though, breaking it up as you go, about 10 minutes. Drain and set aside.

To make the fajitas, add the oil to a medium-size pot over medium-low heat. Add the onion, garlic, salt, pepper, smoked paprika, cumin, and chili powder. Sauté until the onions and garlic are soft, about 5 minutes.

Add the bell peppers and continue to sauté until soft, about 10 minutes. Add the tempeh (or cooked chicken), lime zest, and lime juice. Stir well.

Serve in jicama taco shells, garnished with the avocado and cilantro. Store any leftovers in the fridge in an airtight container for up to 3 days.

butternut scramble over mixed greens

Tofu makes a great swap for eggs, so feel free to use either in any recipe for a scramble! An added bonus in this recipe is butternut squash. It is high in vitamin A, which is great for our mucosal immunity and for regulating blood sugar. It's been used in many countries to control diabetes. Consuming it with balsamic vinegar helps slow the rise in sugar. This is a great choice for your first morning meal.

SERVINGS: 4
PREP TIME: 10 MIN
COOK TIME: 20 MIN

VEGETARIAN
DAIRY-FREE
GLUTEN-FREE
GRAIN-FREE
(VEGAN OPTION)

superfoods used

AVOCADO OIL
ONION
GARLIC
KALE
BUTTERNUT SQUASH
LEMON
OLIVE OIL
TOFU

nutrition info

CALORIES: 326
FAT: 24
CARBS: 10
NET CARBS: 7
FIBER: 3
PROTEIN: 18

nutrition info for vegan option

CALORIES: 304
FAT: 20
CARBS: 11
NET CARBS: 8
FIBER: 3
PROTEIN: 20

BUTTERNUT SQUASH

- 2 tablespoons (30 ml) avocado oil
- 1 teaspoon (6 g) sea salt
- ½ teaspoon (3 g) black pepper
- 3 cups (615 g) cubed butternut squash
- ½ medium (75 g) yellow or red onion, minced
- 3 small (12 g) cloves garlic, minced

MIXED GREENS

- 2 tablespoons (30 ml) olive oil
- 2 tablespoons (30 ml) balsamic vinegar
- 8 cups (360 g) mixed greens, such as kale, spinach, arugula, or radicchio

EGGS

- 8 large eggs (or 14 ounces [400 g] extra-firm tofu)
- 2 tablespoons (10 g) nutritional yeast
- Zest from ½ medium (13 g) fresh lemon

Preheat the oven to 400°F (200°C). Line a baking sheet with parchment paper.

To make the squash, add the oil, salt, and pepper to a large mixing bowl. Add the butternut, onion, and garlic and toss in the oil mixture until everything is coated. Arrange on the prepared baking sheet and bake for 30 minutes, tossing at the halfway mark.

Prepare the mixed greens by adding the olive oil and balsamic vinegar to a large mixing bowl. Whisk well. Add the greens to the bowl and toss until well coated. Set aside.

When the butternut is done, add it to a large skillet over medium-low heat. Crack the eggs directly into the skillet and scramble with the butternut (or crumble in the tofu), keeping the butternut as intact as possible. Season with the nutritional yeast, salt, and pepper.

Remove from the heat and add the lemon zest. Serve over the mixed greens. Store any leftovers in the fridge in an airtight container for up to 3 days.

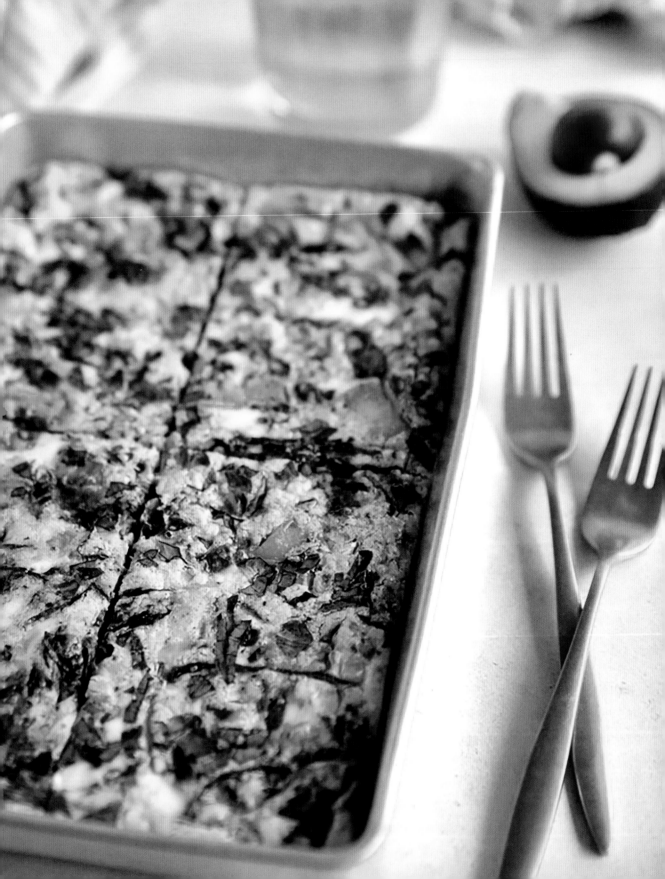

everyday veggie egg bake

This baked egg dish is simple to prepare and easy to reheat throughout the week. You can use any color of bell pepper in the recipe, and use different greens such as kale, arugula, or Swiss chard. Greens provide your body with the micronutrients necessary to support your liver and detoxification processes. You really can't go wrong with which greens you choose—just pick the one you like because you'll be more likely to eat and enjoy them!

SERVINGS: 4
PREP TIME: 10 MIN
COOK TIME: 20 MIN

VEGETARIAN
DAIRY-FREE
GLUTEN-FREE
GRAIN-FREE

VEGETABLES

- 2 tablespoons (30 ml) avocado oil
- ½ medium (75 g) red onion, diced
- 1 medium (150 g) orange bell pepper, seeded and diced
- 1 teaspoon (6 g) sea salt
- ½ teaspoon (3 g) black pepper
- 4 cups (80 g) baby spinach, chopped

EGGS

- 12 large eggs
- 2 tablespoons (10 g) nutritional yeast
- 1 teaspoon (6 g) sea salt
- ½ teaspoon (3 g) black pepper
- 1 medium (150 g) avocado, peeled, pitted, and diced
- ¼ cup (4 g) fresh parsley, basil, or cilantro, minced

Preheat the oven to 400°F (200°C) and grease a 9- x 13-inch (23- x 33-cm) baking pan.

To make the vegetables, add the oil to a large skillet over medium heat. Add the onion and bell pepper and season with the salt and pepper. Sauté until soft, about 5 minutes. Add the baby spinach. Continue to sauté until the spinach has wilted, about 3 minutes. Remove from the heat, drain any excess water, and spread the veggies in the prepared baking pan in an even layer.

To make the eggs, crack the eggs into a large mixing bowl. Add the nutritional yeast, salt, and pepper and whisk to combine. Pour over the veggies. Add the avocado and herbs on top. Bake in the oven until the eggs are set, 15 to 20 minutes.

Remove from the oven and slice into four large squares. Serve and enjoy! Store any leftovers in the fridge in an airtight container for up to 3 days.

superfoods used

AVOCADO OIL
RED ONION
BELL PEPPER
AVOCADO
SPINACH

nutrition info

CALORIES: 379
FAT: 28
CARBS: 8
NET CARBS: 2
FIBER: 2
PROTEIN: 23

egg muffins

with butternut and sunflower seed pesto

SERVINGS: 12
PREP TIME: 10 MIN
COOK TIME: 20 MIN

VEGETARIAN
DAIRY-FREE
GLUTEN-FREE
GRAIN-FREE

I love the combination of creamy butternut and pesto in this recipe. I used sunflower seeds, which are high in vitamin E and magnesium. They provide delicious flavor to these egg muffins. Vitamin E consists of a family of powerful antioxidants. Magnesium is critical for more than 600 enzymatic reactions in the body; several studies have found low magnesium is correlated with high inflammation. These are great to prep early in the week and can be eaten while on the go.

superfoods used

**OLIVE OIL
LEMON
GARLIC
BASIL
SUNFLOWER SEED
AVOCADO OIL
BUTTERNUT SQUASH**

nutrition info

CALORIES: 130
FAT: 10
CARBS: 4
NET CARBS: 2
FIBER: 2
PROTEIN: 6

PESTO

- 2 tablespoons (30 ml) olive oil
- 2 tablespoons (30 ml) fresh lemon juice
- ½ teaspoon (3 g) sea salt
- 2 tablespoons (10 g) nutritional yeast
- 1 small (4 g) clove garlic, minced
- 2 cups (40 g) fresh basil
- ¼ cup (28 g) sunflower seeds

EGG MUFFINS

- 2 tablespoons (30 ml) avocado oil
- 2 cups (410 g) cubed butternut squash
- 1 teaspoon (6 g) sea salt
- ½ teaspoon (3 g) black pepper
- 4 cups (80 g) baby spinach, chopped
- 9 large eggs

Preheat the oven to 400°F (200°C) and line a 12-cup muffin tin with silicone or parchment paper liners.

To make the pesto, add the olive oil, lemon juice, salt, nutritional yeast, and garlic to a food processor. Pulse a few times until everything is well combined. Add the basil and sunflower seeds (in batches if necessary). Continue to pulse until creamy.

To make the egg muffins, add the oil to a large skillet over medium heat. Add the butternut squash and season with the salt and pepper. Sauté until soft, about 5 minutes. Add the spinach and continue to sauté until wilted, about 3 minutes. Remove from the heat. Scoop the vegetables into the lined muffin tin.

Crack the eggs into a large mixing bowl. Whisk well. Fill each muffin cup about three-quarters full. Place a spoonful of pesto in the center of each muffin cup. Bake in the oven until the eggs are set, 15 to 20 minutes.

Remove from the oven and let cool for a few minutes before serving. Store any leftovers in the fridge in an airtight container for up to 3 days.

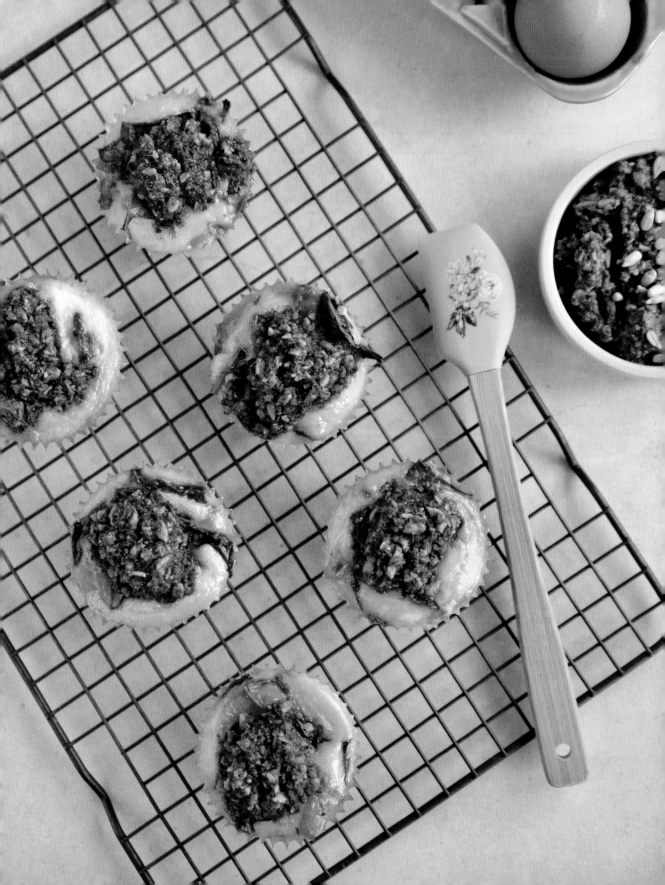

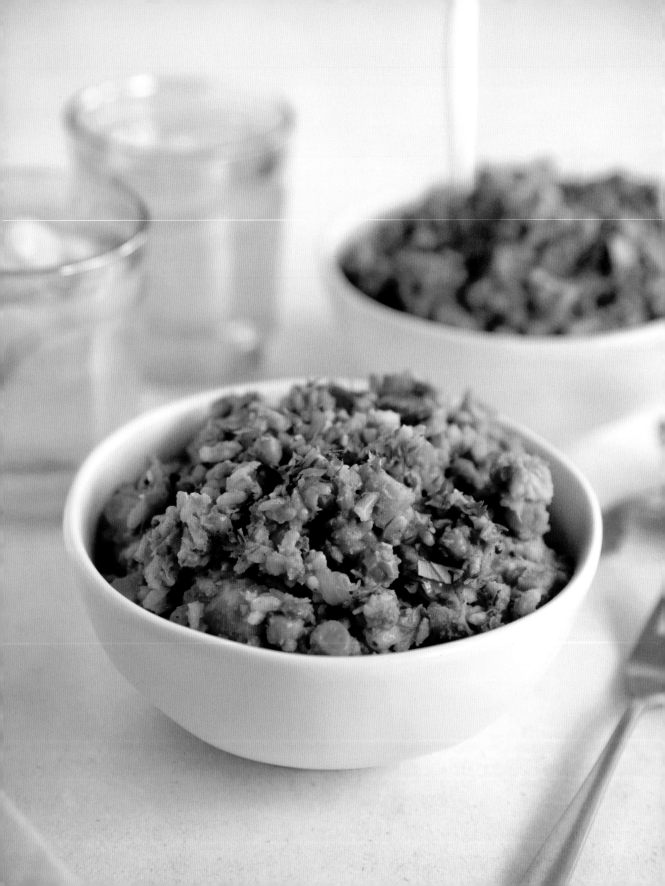

grounding daily kichadi

This ancient Indian dish is cleansing and easy for most people to digest. It is often prepared in a large batch and eaten for several meals in a row. Mustard seed is considered a cruciferous vegetable and has great antioxidant and anti-inflammatory potential. Black cumin seed is known to possess a variety of medicinal activities. This is an excellent, soothing choice for any meal!

SERVINGS: 8
PREP TIME: 15 MIN PLUS SOAKING OVERNIGHT
COOK TIME: 1 HOUR

VEGETARIAN
VEGAN
DAIRY-FREE
GLUTEN-FREE

superfoods used

AVOCADO OIL
BLACK CUMIN SEED
MUSTARD SEED
TOMATO
TURMERIC
CINNAMON
ONION
CARROT
SWEET POTATO
LENTILS
LEMON

nutrition info

CALORIES: 303
FAT: 4
CARBS: 55
NET CARBS: 42
FIBER: 13
PROTEIN: 12

KICHADI

- 1 cup (200 g) brown rice
- 1 cup (200 g) dried brown or green lentils
- 1 tablespoon (15 ml) avocado oil
- 2 teaspoons (4 g) black cumin seeds
- 1 tablespoon (6 g) mustard seeds
- 2 teaspoons (4 g) coriander seeds
- 1 tablespoon (6 g) peeled and grated fresh ginger
- 1 cup (100 g) cherry tomatoes, halved
- 1 cinnamon stick or 2 teaspoons (6 g) ground cinnamon
- 1 teaspoon (5 g) ground turmeric
- 2 medium (300 g) yellow onions, diced
- 2 medium (120 g) carrots, peeled and diced
- 1 medium (130 g) sweet potato, peeled and diced
- 1 teaspoon (6 g) sea salt
- ½ teaspoon (3 g) black pepper
- 4 cups (960 ml) water
- 1 cup (130 g) frozen English peas
- 2 tablespoons (30 ml) fresh lemon juice
- Zest from ½ medium (13 g) fresh lemon

GARNISH

- ½ cup (8 g) fresh cilantro, minced

To make the kichadi, soak the rice and lentils in water to cover for 8 hours or overnight. Drain and rinse very well in a colander. Set aside.

Add the oil to a large pot over medium-low heat. Add the cumin, mustard, and coriander seeds and cook, stirring, until they are toasted and fragrant, about 3 minutes.

Add the ginger, cherry tomatoes, cinnamon, and turmeric and stir to combine. Add the onion, carrots, sweet potato, drained rice and lentils, salt, pepper, and water. Decrease the heat to a simmer and cook for 45 minutes, or until the veggies are soft and the rice and lentils are fluffy and everything has a porridge consistency.

Add the peas and stir until they are defrosted. Stir in the lemon zest and juice. Remove the cinnamon stick, if using. Serve garnished with the cilantro. Store leftovers in the fridge in an airtight container for up to 5 days.

baked oatmeal with mixed berries

SERVINGS: 4
PREP TIME: 10 MIN
COOK TIME: 45 MIN

VEGETARIAN
DAIRY-FREE
GLUTEN-FREE

superfoods used

AVOCADO OIL
CINNAMON
BERRIES
LEMON
HEMP SEED

nutrition info

CALORIES: 443
FAT: 31
CARBS: 28
NET CARBS: 24
FIBER: 4
PROTEIN: 13

Did you know that sprouting oats increases their protein and amino acids? They are high in magnesium and lower in phytates, making them easier to digest and increasing their nutrient bioavailability. You can sprout them yourself by rinsing regular oats of any debris and soaking them in a jar with water for 6 to 12 hours, stirring a few times, and rinsing once more before cooking. Add in those hemp seeds to get more protein, as they contain all nine essential amino acids!

OATMEAL

- 1 teaspoon (5 g) avocado oil to grease baking dish
- 1 cup (90 g) dry sprouted oats
- 1 can (14 ounces, or 400 ml) full-fat coconut milk
- 1 cup (240 ml) plain, unsweetened almond milk or your choice of plant-based milk

  Pinch of sea salt

- 2 teaspoons (6 g) ground cinnamon
- 1 tablespoon (15 g) honey or maple syrup
- 1 teaspoon (4 g) vanilla bean powder
- 4 large eggs, separated
- 1 cup (140 g) fresh mixed berries, chopped if large

  Zest from ½ medium (13 g) fresh lemon

GARNISH

- ½ cup (70 g) fresh mixed berries, chopped
- ¼ cup (18 g) shredded unsweetened coconut, toasted
- 2 tablespoons (20 g) hemp seeds

Preheat the oven to 350°F (175°C) and grease a 2-quart (2-L) baking dish with the oil.

To make the oatmeal, add the sprouted oats, coconut milk, almond milk, salt, and cinnamon to a medium pot over medium-high heat. When it begins to boil, decrease the heat to a simmer. Stir often until the oats are soft and cooked through, having absorbed the liquids, about 15 minutes.

Add the honey and vanilla bean powder. Stir well. Remove from the heat. When it has slightly cooled, mix in the egg yolks.

In a large bowl using an electric mixer, beat the egg whites until stiff peaks have formed, 3 to 5 minutes. Gently fold into the oats. Fold in the berries and zest.

Pour into the greased baking dish and bake in the oven until it is golden and puffy, 20 to 25 minutes.

Serve immediately, garnished with the mixed berries, toasted coconut, and hemp seeds. Store any leftovers in the fridge in an airtight container for up to 5 days.

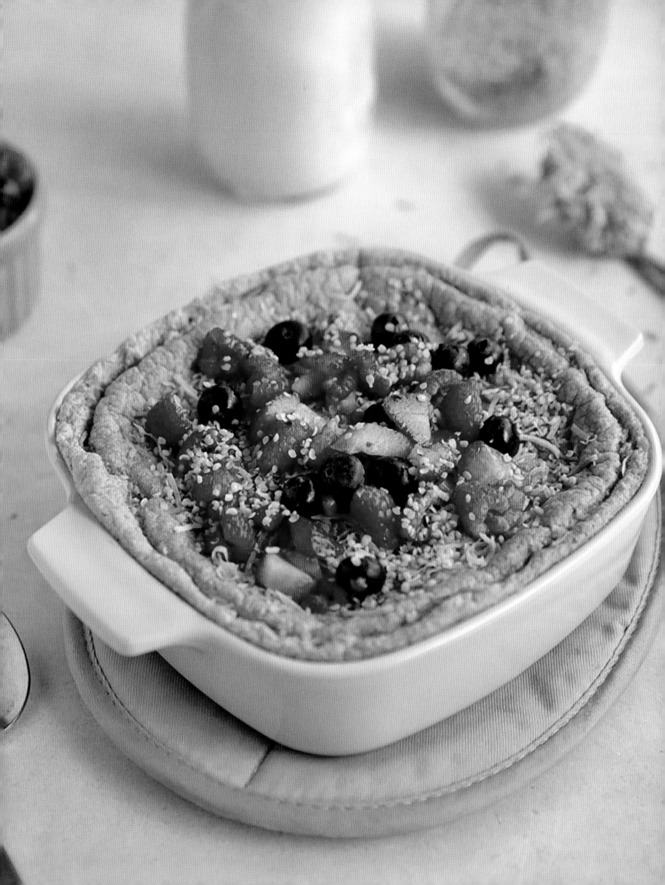

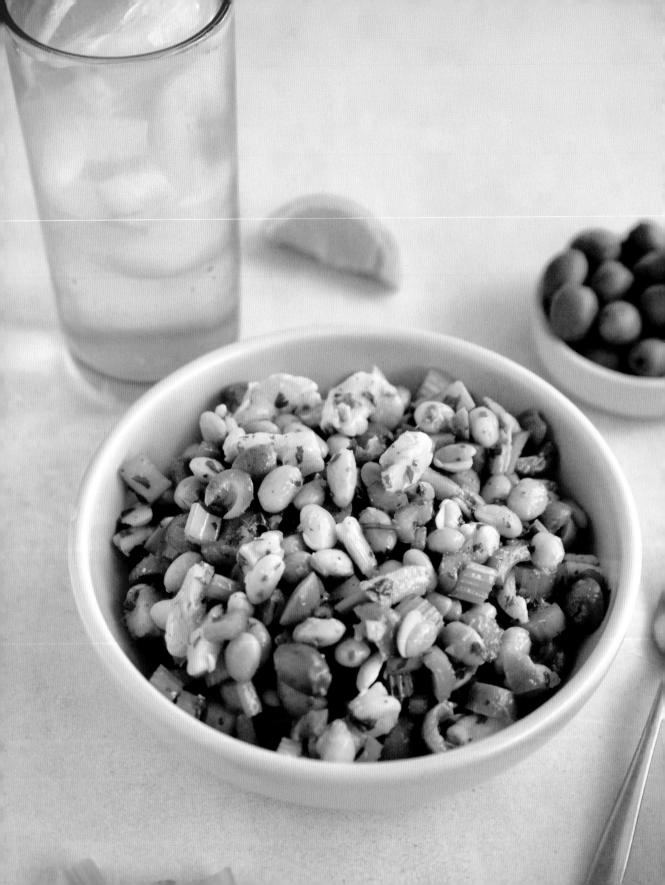

CHAPTER EIGHT

LUNCH

Lunch doesn't have to be another boring salad that gets in all the phytonutrients you need for the day. Boost your immunity and reduce inflammation with lunch recipes your entire family will enjoy. The best part is you can rotate them periodically to keep lunch from getting mundane.

The recipes in this chapter are easy, yet hit all the targets to get your immunity food fix. And while I say you don't want *just another salad*, you will find several salad options that are unique and loaded with antioxidants, vitamins, and minerals. What's even more exciting are the different homemade dressing recipes that you can mix and match with different salad bases and proteins. Not sure where to start? You can't go wrong with the Zoodle Broccoli Bowl with Tempeh and Pesto (page 116) or the Sun-Dried Tomato Pesto Zoodle Bowl (page 115)!

As you scroll through these recipes, don't be afraid to apply what you've learned in the *Immunity Food Fix*. Maybe you want to top off a salad with some sunflower seeds because you are focused on seed cycling for hormones, or maybe add some hemp hearts for extra protein and to reduce inflammation. The beauty of these recipes is you can make them your own. Add in those phytonutrients and get your immunity food fix on!

Citrus Olive Salad with Shrimp,
Edamame, and Cilantro
Vinaigrette, page 128

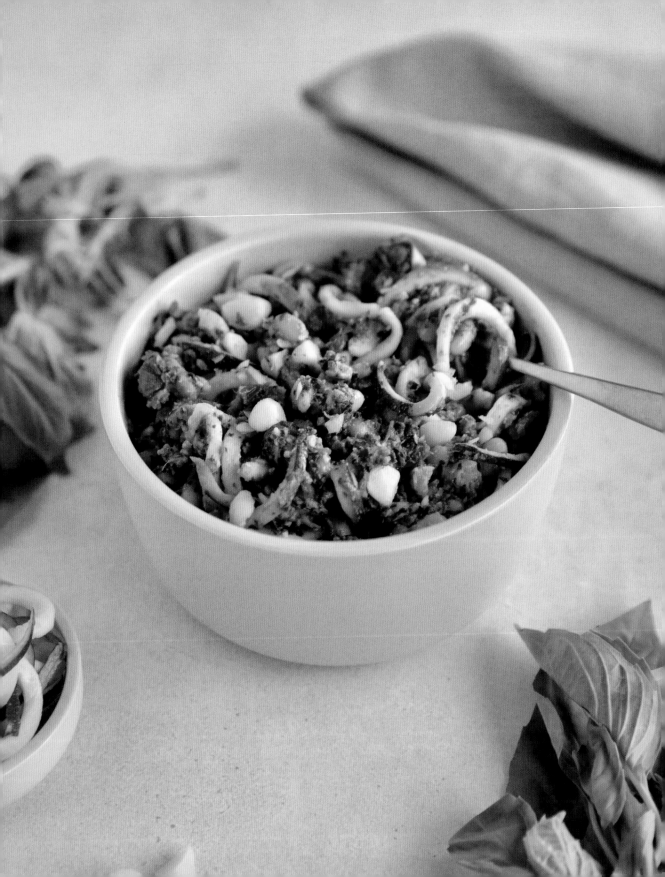

sun-dried tomato pesto zoodle bowl

SERVINGS: 2
PREP TIME: 20 MIN
COOK TIME: 10 MIN

VEGETARIAN
VEGAN
DAIRY-FREE
GLUTEN-FREE
GRAIN-FREE

When shopping for sun-dried tomatoes, make sure they are packed in a healthy oil such as olive oil. Avoid inflammatory oils (such as canola), sulfites, and preservatives. Macadamia nuts give this recipe a creaminess, and macadamias are known to have the highest amount of healthy unsaturated fats among their other nut competitors. They are great for lowering cholesterol and reducing inflammation. This pesto sauce can easily be used on a gluten-free pasta alternative as well. You can easily mix in the zoodles and your kids will never notice!

superfoods used

OLIVE OIL
LEMON
GARLIC
BASIL
MACADAMIA NUT
TOMATO

ZOODLES AND BEANS

- 3 small (369 g) zucchini, ends trimmed
- 1 cup (170 g) cooked white beans

SUN-DRIED TOMATO PESTO

- 2 tablespoons (30 ml) olive oil
- 2 tablespoons (30 ml) fresh lemon juice
- ½ teaspoon (3 g) sea salt
- 2 tablespoons (10 g) nutritional yeast
- 1 small (4 g) clove garlic, minced
- 2 cups (40 g) fresh basil
- ¼ cup (28 g) macadamia nuts
- ½ cup (120 g) julienned sun-dried tomatoes, packed in olive oil

GARNISH

- 2 tablespoons (14 g) macadamia nuts, chopped

nutrition info

CALORIES: 557
FAT: 36
CARBS: 82
NET CARBS: 55
FIBER: 27
PROTEIN: 32

To make the zoodles and beans, use a spiralizer to create zoodles with your zucchini. Set aside. If using canned white beans, drain and rinse them. Add 2 inches (5 cm) of water to a medium pot over high heat. Add the zoodles to a steam basket and steam until soft, about 5 minutes. Set aside.

To make the pesto, add the olive oil, lemon juice, salt, nutritional yeast, and garlic to a food processor. Pulse a few times until everything is well combined. Add the basil, macadamia nuts, and sun-dried tomatoes (in batches if necessary). Continue to pulse until creamy but with a bit of texture. Transfer the pesto to a mixing bowl.

Add the zoodles and white beans to the mixing bowl and gently toss with the pesto until fully coated. Serve garnished with the macadamia nuts. Store any leftovers in the fridge in an airtight container for up to 5 days.

zoodle broccoli bowl

with tempeh and pesto

SERVINGS: 2
PREP TIME: 10 MIN
COOK TIME: 10 MIN

VEGETARIAN
VEGAN
DAIRY-FREE
GLUTEN-FREE
(NON-VEGAN OPTION)

I love the addition of broccoli here, which is excellent to support your liver's detoxification system. Opt for tempeh without added flavoring or preservatives, or you can easily swap it with extra-firm tofu. If plant-based proteins are not your thing, you can't go wrong with ground turkey. If you want to speed this recipe up, many grocery stores sell zucchini spiralized as zoodles in the produce department with the prepackaged leafy greens and vegetables.

superfoods used

BROCCOLI
OLIVE OIL
GARLIC
BASIL
WALNUT
TEMPEH

nutrition info

NUTRITION INFO
CALORIES: 461
FAT: 29
CARBS: 43
NET CARBS: 29
FIBER: 14
PROTEIN: 29

nutrition info for non-vegan option

CALORIES: 502
FAT: 32
CARBS: 22
NET CARBS: 12
FIBER: 10
PROTEIN: 36

PROTEIN

6 ounces (170 g) tempeh, crumbled (or 8 ounces [228 g] ground turkey)

ZOODLE BROCCOLI BOWL

2 small (236 g) zucchini, ends trimmed

2 cups (142 g) broccoli florets

⅔ cup (89 g) frozen English peas

PESTO

2 tablespoons (30 ml) olive oil

2 tablespoons (30 ml) fresh lemon juice

½ teaspoon (3 g) sea salt

2 tablespoons (10 g) nutritional yeast

1 small (4 g) clove garlic, minced

2 cups (40 g) fresh basil

¼ cup (28 g) walnuts

If preparing the non-vegan option, add the turkey to a large, nonstick skillet. Sauté over medium-low heat until fully cooked though, breaking it up as you go, for about 10 minutes. Drain and set aside.

To make the zoodle broccoli bowl, use a spiralizer to create zoodles with your zucchini. Set aside. Add 2 inches (5 cm) of water to a medium pot over high heat. Add the broccoli to a steam basket, followed by the zoodles and English peas. Steam until all the veggies are soft, about 5 minutes. Set aside.

To make the pesto, add the olive oil, lemon juice, salt, nutritional yeast, and garlic to a food processor. Pulse a few times until everything is well combined. Add the basil and walnuts (in batches if necessary). Continue to pulse until creamy.

Add the broccoli, zoodles, and peas to two bowls and garnish with the crumbled tempeh or cooked turkey. Drizzle the pesto over the bowls.

Serve and enjoy! Store any leftovers in the fridge in an airtight container for up to 5 days.

mango salad

with raspberries, beets, and avocado

SERVINGS: 2
PREP TIME: 10 MIN
COOK TIME: 10 MIN

This salad makes eating the rainbow easy, as it contains bright colors from so many fruits and vegetables. Let's talk about the benefits of this combination. With mangos as our base, we know the mangiferin is beneficial to helping regulate blood sugar. Add in those raspberries for gut health and fiber content. The betalains in beets boost our antioxidants. Now top it all off with an avocado—the super fruit full of healthy fat, protein, and, a little hidden secret, FIBER! You know this is an antioxidant powerhouse because it is so colorful!

VEGETARIAN
VEGAN
DAIRY-FREE
GLUTEN-FREE
GRAIN-FREE

superfoods used

OLIVE OIL
ORANGE
MANGO
RASPBERRY
BEET
TOMATO
AVOCADO
WALNUT

MANGO SALAD

- 6½ ounces (200 g) red beets, ends trimmed and peeled
- 1 cup (112 g) chopped fresh mango
- ⅔ cup (82 g) fresh raspberries, halved
- ½ cup (100 g) cherry tomatoes, halved
- 1 medium (150 g) avocado, peeled, pitted, and diced
- ¼ cup (28 g) walnuts, chopped

CINNAMON DIJON VINAIGRETTE

- 3 tablespoons (45 ml) olive oil
- 2 tablespoons (30 ml) fresh orange juice
- 1 tablespoon (15 ml) raw apple cider vinegar
- 1 teaspoon (6 g) sea salt
- ½ teaspoon (3 g) black pepper
- 1 teaspoon (3 g) ground cinnamon
- 1 teaspoon (5 g) Dijon mustard

To make the mango salad, add 2 inches (5 cm) of water to a medium pot on the stove and place over high heat. Chop the beets in 1" pieces and add them to a steam basket and steam until soft, 8 to 10 minutes. Set aside.

To make the vinaigrette, add all the ingredients to a mixing bowl and whisk until well combined. Set aside.

To finish the salad, add the salad ingredients to the bowl of vinaigrette and gently toss until everything is coated. Serve and enjoy! Store any leftovers in the fridge in an airtight container for up to 5 days.

nutrition info

CALORIES: 493
FAT: 37
CARBS: 38
NET CARBS: 24
FIBER: 14
PROTEIN: 6

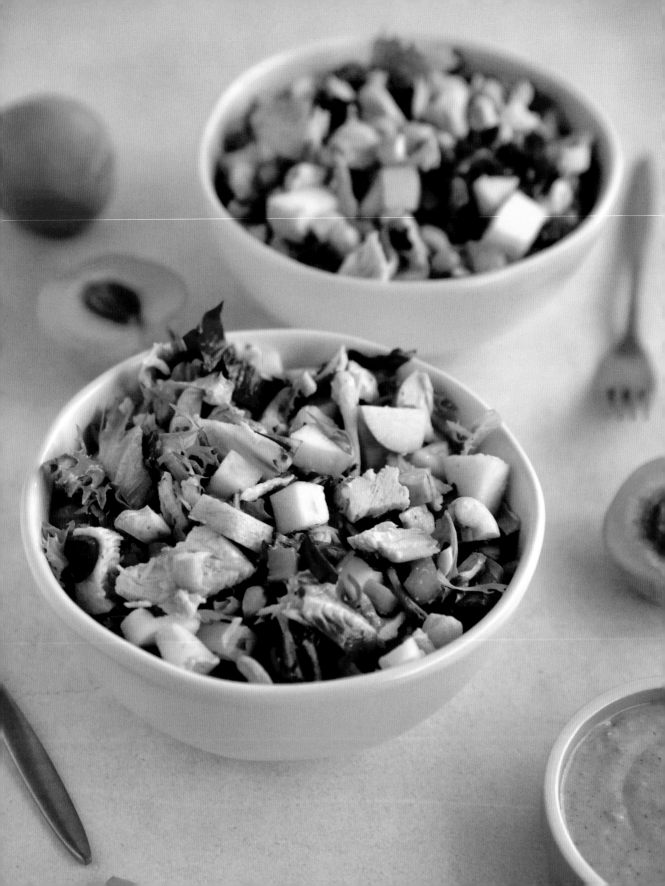

chicken radicchio salad with apple, celery, and cashews

with apricot dressing

SERVINGS: 2
PREP TIME: 15 MIN
COOK TIME: 0 MIN

DAIRY-FREE
GLUTEN-FREE
GRAIN-FREE
(VEGAN OPTION)

Blending apricot into your dressing amps up its flavor and nutrition. Apricots are rich in vitamin A, providing you 20 percent of your RDA in just one fruit. Vitamin A is important for our immune system and increasing IgA levels. Apricots are naturally sweet; no added sugars are necessary to create a delicious dressing for this salad. Celery is also a bonus for our gut lining. Let's not forget the benefits of the pectin fibers in apples, putting us in an anti-inflammatory state. Just remember not to remove the skin!

superfoods used

OLIVE OIL
SESAME SEED
LEMON
APRICOT
CELERY
APPLE
AVOCADO
CASHEW
CHICKPEA

APRICOT DRESSING

- 2 tablespoons (30 ml) olive oil
- 2 tablespoons (30 g) tahini
- 2 tablespoons (30 ml) fresh lemon juice
- 1 tablespoon (15 ml) raw apple cider vinegar
- 1 teaspoon (6 g) sea salt
- ½ teaspoon (3 g) black pepper
- 1 teaspoon (3 g) ground cinnamon
- 1 (35 g) ripe apricot, pitted and chopped

CHICKEN SALAD

- 1½ cups (210 g) chopped boneless, skinless chicken breast (or 6 ounces [170 g] cooked chickpeas)
- 2 cups (85 g) radicchio, chopped
- 2 cups (85 g) mixed greens, such as kale, spinach, arugula, or butter lettuce
- 2 medium (115 g) apples, cored and diced
- 1 cup (100 g) diced celery
- 1 tablespoon (10 g) minced shallot
- ½ medium (75 g) avocado, peeled, pitted, and diced
- 2 tablespoons (14 g) chopped cashews

To make the dressing, add all the ingredients to a blender. Blend on high speed until very creamy, scraping down the sides of the blender as needed. If it is too thick for your preference, add 1 tablespoon (15 ml) of water and blend again, repeating until it is to your liking. Pour into a large mixing bowl.

To make the chicken salad, add all the ingredients to the mixing bowl and gently stir until coated. Serve and enjoy! Store any leftovers in the fridge in an airtight container for up to 3 days.

nutrition info

CALORIES: 542
FAT: 32
CARBS: 22
NET CARBS: 14
FIBER: 8
PROTEIN: 38

nutrition info for vegan option

CALORIES: 510
FAT: 31
CARBS: 45
NET CARBS: 30
FIBER: 15
PROTEIN: 14

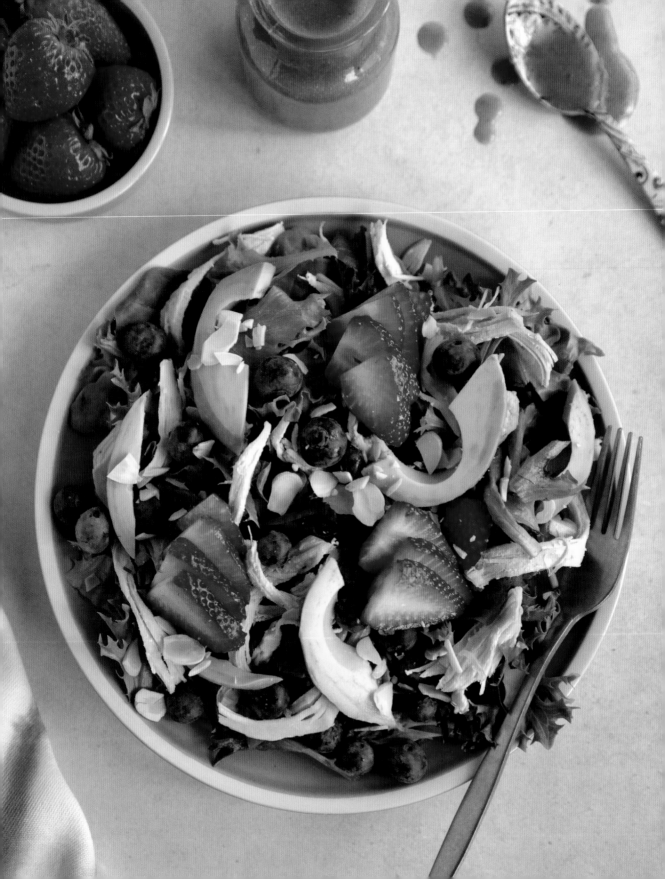

chicken and kale salad with berries and strawberry-balsamic vinaigrette

SERVINGS: 2
PREP TIME: 15 MIN
COOK TIME: 0 MIN

DAIRY-FREE
GLUTEN-FREE
GRAIN-FREE
(VEGAN OPTION)

This colorful salad is bursting with fresh flavor and loaded with antioxidants, vitamins, and minerals. If you cannot source blueberries, you can replace them with raspberries, blackberries, or grapes. This recipe contains four cups of your favorite greens, and you can easily add more and mix and match. Kale, spinach, and arugula all have detoxification properties to support our liver. Kale, being part of the brassica family of vegetables like broccoli and cauliflower, is a great source of prebiotic fibers, supporting your gut microbiome.

superfoods used

OLIVE OIL
ORANGE
KALE
BLUEBERRY
AVOCADO
ALMOND

STRAWBERRY-BALSAMIC VINAIGRETTE

- 2 tablespoons (30 ml) olive oil
- 2 tablespoons (30 ml) fresh orange juice
- 2 teaspoons (10 ml) balsamic vinegar
- 1 teaspoon (6 g) sea salt
- ½ teaspoon (3 g) black pepper
- ¼ cup (43 g) sliced strawberries

CHICKEN SPINACH SALAD

- 1½ cups (210 g) chopped boneless, skinless chicken breast (or 1½ cups [234 g] shelled edamame)
- 2 cups (85 g) baby spinach
- 2 cups (85 g) mixed greens such as kale, spinach, arugula, or butter lettuce
- 1 cup (166 g) sliced strawberries
- ½ cup (48 g) blueberries
- 1 tablespoon (10 g) minced shallot
- 1 medium (150 g) avocado, peeled, pitted, and diced
- 2 tablespoons (14 g) sliced almonds

To make the vinaigrette, add all the ingredients to a blender. Blend on high speed until very creamy, scraping down the sides of the blender as needed. If it is too thick for your preference, add 1 tablespoon (15 ml) of water and blend again, repeating until it is to your liking. Pour into a large mixing bowl.

To make the salad, add all the ingredients to the mixing bowl. Gently toss until coated. Serve and enjoy! Store any leftovers in the fridge in an airtight container for up to 3 days.

nutrition info

CALORIES: 552
FAT: 33
CARBS: 21
NET CARBS: 11
FIBER: 10
PROTEIN: 38

nutrition info for vegan option

CALORIES: 536
FAT: 34
CARBS: 33
NET CARBS: 21
FIBER: 12
PROTEIN: 19

chicken-avocado waldorf salad

SERVINGS: 2
PREP TIME: 15 MIN
COOK TIME: 0 MIN

DAIRY-FREE
GLUTEN-FREE
GRAIN-FREE
(VEGAN OPTION)

superfoods used

AVOCADO
OLIVE OIL
SESAME SEED
LEMON
APPLE
CELERY
WALNUT

nutrition info

CALORIES: 526
FAT: 31
CARBS: 26
NET CARBS: 16
FIBER: 10
PROTEIN: 36

*nutrition info for
vegan option*

CALORIES: 496
FAT: 30
CARBS: 47
NET CARBS: 32
FIBER: 15
PROTEIN: 12

This recipe is a twist on your typical chicken salad, and the secret is in the dressing. Avocado and tahini create a creamy dressing for this classic, and the combination of the sesame seeds and avocado give you an excellent phytonutrient profile that is both anti-inflammatory and immune modulating. They also add healthy fats that allow you to absorb the vitamins in this delicious recipe and give you that satiety you need in the middle of the day!

DRESSING

- 1 medium (150 g) avocado, peeled, pitted, and chopped
- 1 tablespoon (15 ml) olive oil
- 1 tablespoon (15 g) tahini
- 1 tablespoon (15 ml) fresh lemon juice
- 1 teaspoon (6 g) sea salt
- ½ teaspoon (3 g) black pepper

SALAD

- 1½ cups (210 g) chopped boneless, skinless chicken breast (or 1 cup [170 g] cooked chickpeas)
- 1 medium (115 g) apple, cored and diced
- ½ cup (75 g) grapes, halved
- ½ cup (50 g) diced celery
- 1 tablespoon (10 g) minced shallot
- ¼ cup (28 g) chopped walnuts
- Salad greens (optional)

To make the dressing, add all the ingredients to a food processor and pulse until very creamy, scraping down the sides of the bowl as needed. Pour into a large mixing bowl.

To make the salad, add all the ingredients to the mixing bowl. Gently stir until coated.

Serve as is or over a bed of leafy greens. Store any leftovers in the fridge in an airtight container for up to 3 days.

tuna, chickpea, and arugula salad

with lemon and tarragon vinaigrette

SERVINGS: 2
PREP TIME: 15 MIN
COOK TIME: 0 MIN

DAIRY-FREE
GLUTEN-FREE
GRAIN-FREE
(VEGAN OPTION)

Canned tuna makes a fast protein option, and it is high in vitamin D, which promotes healthy bones and strengthens the immune system. This recipe helps you add color and nutrients to that can of tuna. Celery is a common addition in tuna salads. What is surprising is that celery contains the compound apiin, which provides anti-inflammatory benefits. The pectin in celery, similar to apples, is also a great source of fiber, adding to that anti-inflammatory mechanism and improving gut health.

superfoods used

OLIVE OIL
LEMON
CHICKPEA
CELERY
BLUEBERRY
AVOCADO
WALNUT

LEMON TARRAGON VINAIGRETTE

- 2 tablespoons (30 ml) olive oil
- 2 tablespoons (30 ml) fresh lemon juice
- 1 teaspoon (6 g) sea salt
- ½ teaspoon (3 g) black pepper
- 1 teaspoon (1 g) dried tarragon

TUNA, CHICKPEA, AND ARUGULA SALAD

- 1 can (6.4 ounces, or 182 g) chunk light tuna packed in water, drained (or 6 ounces [170 g] crumbled tempeh)
- 1 cup (170 g) cooked chickpeas, drained
- ½ cup (50 g) diced celery
- ½ cup (48 g) blueberries
- 1 medium (150 g) avocado, peeled, pitted, and diced
- 2 tablespoons (14 g) chopped walnuts
- 4 cups (80 g) arugula

To make the vinaigrette, add all the ingredients to a mixing bowl. Whisk together.

To make the salad, add all the ingredients to the mixing bowl. Toss gently until coated.

Serve and enjoy! Store any leftovers in the fridge in an airtight container for up to 2 days.

nutrition info

CALORIES: 427
FAT: 23
CARBS: 32
NET CARBS: 24
FIBER: 8
PROTEIN: 25

nutrition info for vegan option

CALORIES: 426
FAT: 22
CARBS: 53
NET CARBS: 40
FIBER: 13
PROTEIN: 25

roasted fennel and cherry tomatoes

with smoked salmon

DAIRY-FREE
GLUTEN-FREE
GRAIN-FREE
(VEGAN OPTION)

superfoods used

AVOCADO
LEMON
FENNEL
TOMATO
CHICKPEA
SALMON

nutrition info

CALORIES: 500
FAT: 26
CARBS: 37
NET CARBS: 26
FIBER: 11
PROTEIN: 32

nutrition info for vegan option

CALORIES: 447
FAT: 22
CARBS: 58
NET CARBS: 43
FIBER: 15
PROTEIN: 26

Fennel has a sweet flavor with hints of licorice, yet it is also known for cleansing the breath. It tastes amazing with cherry tomatoes, balsamic vinegar, and savory, salty smoked salmon. Fennel is well known for its beneficial effects on digestion and settling the stomach, but it also contains twenty-one fatty acids, which contribute to its anti-inflammatory properties. Chickpeas are an added bonus, being both high in protein and fiber. This is a delicious recipe for any meal of the day!

DRESSING

- 2 tablespoons (30 ml) avocado oil
- 2 tablespoons (30 ml) fresh lemon juice
- 1 tablespoon (15 ml) balsamic vinegar
- 1 teaspoon (6 g) sea salt
- ½ teaspoon (3 g) black pepper

FENNEL SALAD

- 2 cups (180 g) chopped fennel
- 2 cups (200 g) cherry tomatoes
- 6 ounces (170 g) wild smoked salmon (or 6 ounces [170 g] crumbled tempeh)
- 1 cup (170 g) cooked chickpeas, drained

Preheat the oven to 400°F (200°C). Line a baking sheet with parchment paper.

To make the dressing, add all the ingredients to a mixing bowl. Whisk to combine.

Add the fennel and cherry tomatoes to the bowl and toss to coat. Spread in an even layer on the prepared baking sheet and roast in the oven for 25 minutes, tossing at the halfway mark. The fennel will be browned and the cherry tomatoes will be blistered when done.

Remove from the oven and serve with the smoked salmon (or crumbled tempeh) and chickpeas. Store any leftovers in the fridge in an airtight container for up to 2 days.

kohlrabi and apple slaw with tuna

SERVINGS: 2
PREP TIME: 15 MIN
COOK TIME: 0 MIN

DAIRY-FREE
GLUTEN-FREE
GRAIN-FREE
(VEGAN OPTION)

Kohlrabi is a great source of fiber, calcium, and magnesium. It is often enjoyed raw, such as in this recipe, giving it that added crunch. It can be roasted but can get mushy; if you roast it, roast it at a high temperature for a short time. Kohlrabi contains a hidden secret—melatonin! While we typically think of melatonin for sleep, it is essential for the immune system, not only balancing it but also blocking the release of inflammatory cytokines.

SLAW

- 2 tablespoons (30 ml) olive oil
- Zest from ½ medium (13 g) fresh lemon
- 1 tablespoon (15 ml) fresh lemon juice
- 1 teaspoon (6 g) sea salt
- ½ teaspoon (3 g) black pepper
- 1 teaspoon (0.6 g) dried tarragon
- 1 tablespoon (10 g) minced shallot
- 1 medium (15 g) scallion, minced
- ¼ cup (4 g) fresh parsley, minced
- 2 cups (180 g) peeled and shredded/julienned kohlrabi
- 1 medium (80 g) carrot, shredded or julienned
- 1 medium (115 g) apple, cored and julienned
- 1 can (5 ounces, or 142 g) chunk light tuna packed in water, drained (or 5 ounces [142 g] crumbled tempeh)
- 1 medium (150 g) avocado, peeled, pitted, and diced

To make the slaw, in a large bowl, add the olive oil and lemon zest and juice. Whisk well. Season with the salt, pepper, and dried tarragon. Add the shallot, scallion, and parsley. Stir together. Add the kohlrabi, carrot, and apple. Gently toss until coated. Add the tuna (or crumbled tempeh) and avocado. Gently toss together until well combined.

Serve and enjoy! Store any leftovers in the fridge in an airtight container for up to 2 days or 5 days if serving the vegan option.

superfoods used

**OLIVE OIL
LEMON
ONION
KOHLRABI
CARROT
APPLE
TEMPEH
AVOCADO**

nutrition info

**CALORIES: 449
FAT: 28
CARBS: 27
NET CARBS: 14
FIBER: 13
PROTEIN: 22**

nutrition info for vegan option

**CALORIES: 456
FAT: 30
CARBS: 45
NET CARBS: 29
FIBER: 16
PROTEIN: 18**

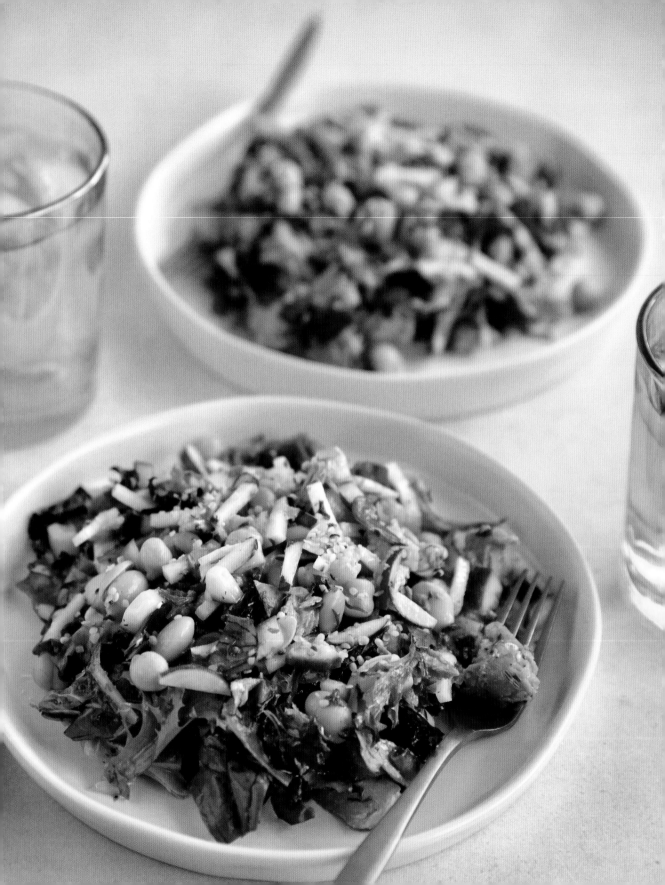

chickpea, edamame, and salmon salad

with lemon basil-dill vinaigrette

SERVINGS: 2
PREP TIME: 15 MIN
COOK TIME: 0 MIN

DAIRY-FREE
GLUTEN-FREE
GRAIN-FREE
(VEGAN OPTION)

Even those who do not like salads will love this one! Creamy and crunchy with loads of flavor from fresh herbs, this is a crowd-pleaser. The edamame provides the body with protein and fiber, but it's also a great source of copper, which is essential for our immune system. Be aware that edamame is tricky for some who can't tolerate soy or respond poorly to increased estrogen. If making a day in advance of eating, toss the salmon in just before serving.

superfoods used

OLIVE OIL
LEMON
BASIL
CHICKPEA
EDAMAME
RADISH
CUCUMBER
HEMP SEED
SALMON

LEMON BASIL-DILL VINAIGRETTE

- 2 tablespoons (30 ml) olive oil
- 2 tablespoons (30 ml) fresh lemon juice
- 1 tablespoon (15 ml) raw apple cider vinegar
- 1 teaspoon (6 g) sea salt
- ½ teaspoon (3 g) black pepper
- 1 tablespoon (3 g) fresh dill, minced
- 1 tablespoon (1 g) fresh basil, minced
- 1 tablespoon (7 g) capers, drained

CHICKPEA, EDAMAME, AND SALMON SALAD

- 1 cup (170 g) cooked chickpeas
- ½ cup (80 g) shelled edamame (or 1 cup [156 g] for vegan option)
- 4 ounces (144 g) cooked skinless salmon, skin removed and chopped (omit for vegan option)
- 4 cups (200 g) mixed greens, such as kale, spinach, arugula, or butter lettuce
- ½ cup (66 g) minced radish
- ½ cup (60 g) diced cucumber
- 1 tablespoon (30 g) hemp seeds

To make the vinaigrette, add all the ingredients to a mixing bowl. Whisk until well combined.

To make the salad, add all the ingredients to the mixing bowl. Toss gently until coated.

Serve and enjoy! Store any leftovers in the fridge in an airtight container for up to 2 days or 5 days if serving the vegan option.

nutrition info

CALORIES: 572
FAT: 31
CARBS: 41
NET CARBS: 30
FIBER: 11
PROTEIN: 33

nutrition info for vegan option

CALORIES: 504
FAT: 25
CARBS: 45
NET CARBS: 34
FIBER: 11
PROTEIN: 26

citrus olive salad

with shrimp, edamame, and cilantro vinaigrette

SERVINGS: 2
PREP TIME: 20 MIN
COOK TIME: 0 MIN

DAIRY-FREE
GLUTEN-FREE
GRAIN-FREE
(VEGAN OPTION)

superfoods used

OLIVE OIL
ORANGE
LEMON
BASIL
AVOCADO OIL
EDAMAME
CELERY

nutrition info

CALORIES: 484
FAT: 38
CARBS: 16
NET CARBS: 14
FIBER: 12
PROTEIN: 21

nutrition info for vegan option

CALORIES: 467
FAT: 39
CARBS: 20
NET CARBS: 18
FIBER: 19
PROTEIN: 12

Pairing tangy, creamy olives and edamame with a bright dressing, crunchy celery, and salty shrimp is a delicious way to eat your vitamins and minerals! Olive oil and avocado oil are my go-to oils because of their polyphenol content and high levels of MUFAs. Both are highly anti-inflammatory and possess beneficial effects on our gut bacteria. The vinaigrette contains cilantro, which aids detoxication, helping to remove heavy metals from the body, and also contains cineole and linoleic acid, which give it its anti-inflammatory properties.

CILANTRO VINAIGRETTE

- 2 tablespoons (30 ml) olive oil
- 2 tablespoons (30 ml) fresh orange juice
- 1 tablespoon (15 ml) fresh lemon juice
- 1 teaspoon (6 g) sea salt
- ½ teaspoon (3 g) black pepper
- ¼ cup (4 g) fresh cilantro
- ¼ cup (4 g) fresh basil
- ¼ cup (28 g) pine nuts

SHRIMP

- 1 teaspoon (5 ml) avocado oil
- 4 ounces (144 g) shrimp, deveined and tails removed (omit for vegan option)
- ½ teaspoon (3 g) sea salt
- ¼ teaspoon (2 g) black pepper

SALAD

- ½ cup (90 g) green olives, pitted and chopped
- ½ cup (80 g) shelled edamame (or 1 cup [156 g] for vegan option)
- 1 cup (100 g) diced celery

To make the vinaigrette, add all the ingredients to a blender. Blend on high speed until very creamy, scraping down the sides of the blender as needed. If it is too thick for your preference, add 1 tablespoon (15 ml) of water and blend again, repeating until it is to your liking. Pour into a large mixing bowl.

To make the shrimp, add the oil to a large, cast-iron skillet over medium-high heat. When hot, place the shrimp in the skillet and do not move. Season with the salt and pepper and sear on each side for 2 minutes. Remove from the heat and set aside to cool. When cool, chop into small pieces.

To make the salad, add all the ingredients, including the shrimp, to the mixing bowl. Toss gently until coated.

Serve and enjoy! Store any leftovers in the fridge in an airtight container for up to 2 days or 5 days if serving the vegan option.

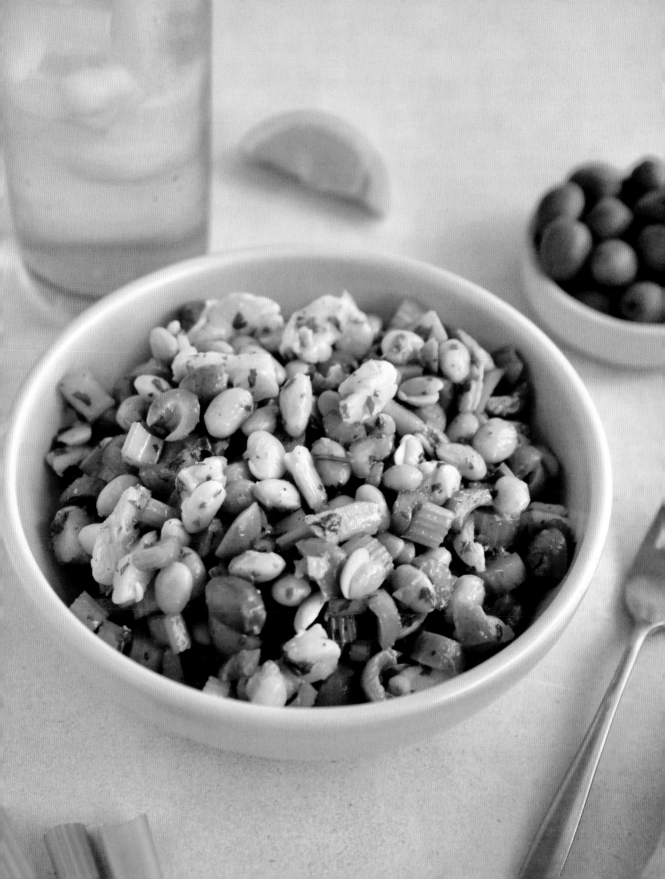

cabbage salad lettuce wraps with spicy chicken

SERVINGS: 2
PREP TIME: 20 MIN
COOK TIME: 0 MIN

DAIRY-FREE
GLUTEN-FREE
GRAIN-FREE
(VEGAN OPTION)

superfoods used

**SESAME OIL
LIME
CARROT
PUMPKIN SEED
CABBAGE**

nutrition info

**CALORIES: 384
FAT: 18
CARBS: 11
NET CARBS: 8
FIBER: 3
PROTEIN: 33**

*nutrition info for
vegan option*

**CALORIES: 368
FAT: 21
CARBS: 39
NET CARBS: 31
FIBER: 8
PROTEIN: 23**

Boston lettuce (also called butter or Bibb lettuce) is a great alternative to grain-based wraps. You can find it in the refrigerated section of the produce department in most grocery stores. It is high in vitamins A, C, and K and rich in calcium and iron. Adding cabbage to this recipe gives it its detox boost. Cabbage is part of the brassica family of vegetables and has a beneficial effect on the liver both in phase I and phase II, helping to clear out foreign toxins.

CABBAGE SALAD

- 2 tablespoons (30 ml) sesame oil
- 1 tablespoon (15 ml) coconut aminos

  Zest from ½ medium (11 g) fresh lime
- 1 tablespoon (15 ml) fresh lime juice
- 1 teaspoon (6 g) sea salt
- ½ teaspoon (3 g) black pepper
- 1 tablespoon (10 g) minced shallot
- ¼ cup (4 g) fresh cilantro, minced
- 1 medium scallion (15 g), minced
- 2 cups (180 g) shredded green or purple cabbage
- 1 medium (80 g) carrot, shredded
- ¼ cup (28 g) pepitas

CHICKEN OR TEMPEH

- 8 ounces (228 g) cooked boneless, skinless chicken breast, shredded (or 8 ounces [228 g] crumbled tempeh)
- 2 tablespoons (30 ml) hot sauce
- ½ teaspoon (3 g) sea salt
- ¼ teaspoon (2 g) black pepper

LETTUCE WRAPS

- 1 head Boston lettuce, leaves separated

To make the cabbage salad, in a large bowl, add the sesame oil, coconut aminos, and lime zest and juice. Whisk well. Season with the salt and pepper. Add the shallot, cilantro, and scallion. Stir together. Add the cabbage, carrot, and pepitas and toss gently to coat.

To make the chicken, in a separate mixing bowl, toss together the chicken (or crumbled tempeh), hot sauce, salt, and pepper.

To make the lettuce wraps, fill Boston lettuce leaves with the cabbage salad and spicy chicken (or tempeh). Serve and enjoy! Store any leftovers in the fridge in an airtight container for up to 3 days or 5 days if serving the vegan option.

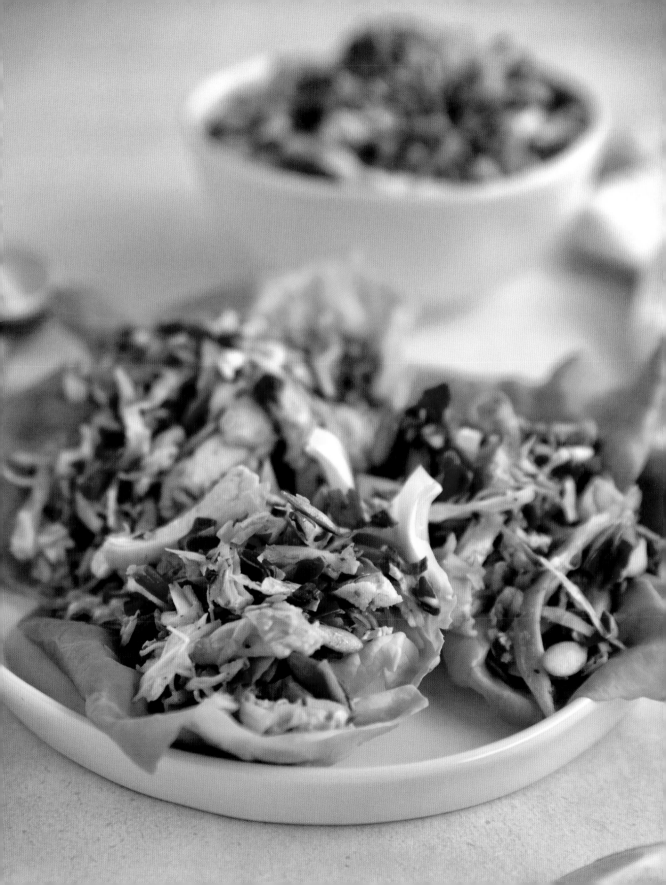

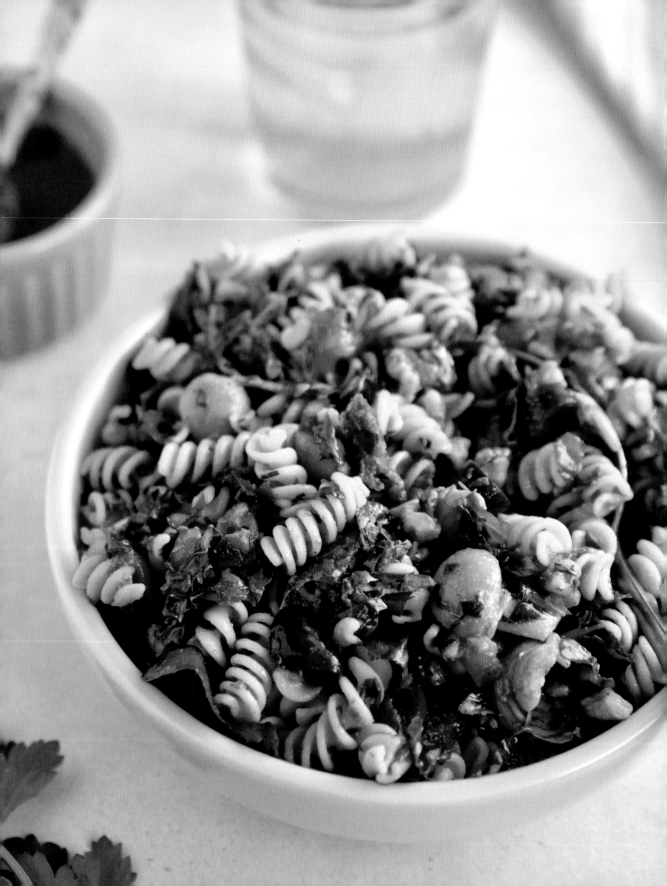

antioxidant-packed antipasto salad

This pasta is perfect to prepare and pack for lunch, whether that is at the office, out on a trail, or simply at home. Increase its protein content by adding chicken breast or tofu. This recipe will last day after day, and it only gets better as the flavors marinate together. When you think antioxidant boost, think of all the different colors of the rainbow you get in just a few bites. This recipe alone is packed with all the plant-based foods you need to hit that target nine to twelve servings!

SERVINGS: 4
PREP TIME: 15 MIN
COOK TIME: 10 MIN

DAIRY-FREE
GLUTEN-FREE
VEGAN
VEGETARIAN

superfoods used

CHICKPEA
OLIVE OIL
KALE
TOMATO
RED PEPPER
LEMON
BASIL
WALNUT

nutrition info

CALORIES: 487
FAT: 28
CARBS: 50
NET CARBS: 40
FIBER: 10
PROTEIN: 16

SALAD

- 8 ounces (228 g) chickpea pasta
- ¼ cup (60 ml) olive oil
- 2 tablespoons (20 g) sliced shallot
- 2 small (8 g) cloves garlic, minced
- 1 teaspoon (6 g) sea salt
- ½ teaspoon (3 g) black pepper
- 4 cups (120 g) baby kale
- ¼ cup (60 g) julienned sun-dried tomatoes, packed in olive oil
- 20 (60 g) pitted kalamata olives, halved
- 2 ounces (60 g) marinated mushrooms, halved
- 1 can (14 ounces, or 240 g) quartered artichoke hearts, drained
- 2 ounces (60 g) jarred roasted red peppers, drained and chopped
- Zest from 1 medium (13 g) fresh lemon
- 2 tablespoons (30 ml) fresh lemon juice
- ¼ cup (4 g) fresh parsley, minced
- ¼ cup (4 g) fresh basil, minced
- ¼ cup (28 g) chopped walnuts

To make the salad, bring a large pot of water to a boil. When boiling, add the chickpea pasta and cook according to package instructions (5 to 10 minutes). When it reaches your desired tenderness, remove from the heat and drain in a colander. Add to a large mixing bowl and set in the fridge to completely cool.

While the pasta is cooking, add the remaining ingredients to a large mixing bowl and gently toss together.

When the pasta is cool, add to it the antipasto bowl and toss together. Serve and enjoy! Store any leftovers in the fridge in an airtight container for up to 5 days.

kale salad with chicken

and sweet chlorella dressing

SERVINGS: 4
PREP TIME: 15 MIN
COOK TIME: 0 MIN

DAIRY-FREE
GLUTEN-FREE
GRAIN-FREE
(VEGAN OPTION)

superfoods used

OLIVE OIL
SESAME SEED
CHLORELLA
KALE
CHICKPEA
APPLE
PUMPKIN SEED
PEPPERMINT

nutrition info

CALORIES: 350
FAT: 17
CARBS: 27
NET CARBS: 21
FIBER: 6
PROTEIN: 22

*nutrition info for
vegan option*

CALORIES: 355
FAT: 18
CARBS: 33
NET CARBS: 26
FIBER: 7
PROTEIN: 15

Did you know chlorella is good for skin health? It helps reduce inflammation and restore the production of collagen. While chlorella isn't necessarily sweet, combining it with maple syrup in this recipe makes it much more palatable without losing any of its benefits. Being a microalga, it's packed with vitamins and minerals, with selenium being in great abundance. Selenium is an excellent antioxidant and important for thyroid health. Adding it to a vinaigrette or dressing is a great way to include this superfood in your diet!

SWEET CHLORELLA DRESSING

- 2 tablespoons (30 ml) olive oil
- 2 tablespoons (30 ml) raw apple cider vinegar
- 2 tablespoons (30 g) tahini
- 1 tablespoon (15 ml) maple syrup
- 1 teaspoon (6 g) sea salt
- ½ teaspoon (3 g) black pepper
- 1 teaspoon (3 g) chlorella powder

KALE SALAD WITH CHICKEN

- 1½ cups (210 g) chopped boneless, skinless chicken breast (or 1½ cups [234 g] shelled edamame)
- 4 cups (400 g) dinosaur kale, stems removed
- 1 cup (170 g) cooked chickpeas, rinsed
- 1 medium (115 g) apple, cored and diced
- ¼ cup (28 g) pepitas
- 4 fresh peppermint leaves, minced

To make the vinaigrette, add all the ingredients to a blender. Blend on high speed until very creamy, scraping down the sides of the blender as needed. If it is too thick for your preference, add 1 tablespoon (15 ml) of water and blend again, repeating until it is to your liking. Pour into a large mixing bowl.

To make the salad, add all the ingredients to the mixing bowl. Toss gently until coated.

Serve and enjoy! Store any leftovers in the fridge in an airtight container for up to 3 days.

roasted cauliflower and chickpeas with cashews

SERVINGS: 4
PREP TIME: 10 MIN
PLUS SOAKING
OVERNIGHT
COOK TIME: 25 MIN

VEGETARIAN
VEGAN
DAIRY-FREE
GLUTEN-FREE

The cashews in this recipe give it a tasty crunch in every bite, but they also have important health benefits! Cashews contain a high amount of phytosterols, which help inhibit cholesterol absorption in the small intestine. They are wonderful eaten raw, or you can toast them on a baking sheet in the oven set to 350°F (175°C) for 8 to 10 minutes, tossing every 3 minutes. Combining these benefits with protein-packed chickpeas and detoxing cauliflower really takes this recipe to the next level.

superfoods used

AVOCADO OIL
LEMON
ONION
CHICKPEA
CASHEW
CAULIFLOWER

CAULIFLOWER AND CHICKPEAS

- 2 tablespoons (30 ml) avocado oil
- 1 tablespoon (15 ml) fresh lemon juice
- 1 teaspoon (6 g) sea salt
- ½ teaspoon (3 g) black pepper
- 4 cups (400 g) cauliflower florets, chopped
- 1 medium (40 g) shallot, minced
- 1 small (4 g) clove garlic, minced
- 15 ounces (425 g) cooked chickpeas, rinsed
- 4 cups (170 g) baby spinach, chopped
- ¼ cup (4 g) fresh parsley or cilantro, minced
- 1 medium (15 g) scallion, minced

GARNISH

- ¼ cup (28 g) cashews, chopped

Preheat the oven to 425°F (220°C). Line a baking sheet with parchment paper.

To make the cauliflower and chickpeas, add the oil, lemon juice, salt, and pepper to a mixing bowl. Stir together. Add the cauliflower florets, shallot, garlic, and chickpeas to the bowl and gently toss until everything is coated.

Spread in an even layer on the prepared baking sheet and bake in the oven for 20 minutes, tossing at the halfway mark. When there are 5 minutes left, add the baby spinach to the baking sheet, toss together, and let it wilt. Remove from the oven and stir in the parsley and scallion.

Serve garnished with the cashews. Store any leftovers in the fridge in an airtight container for up to 5 days.

nutrition info

CALORIES: 293
FAT: 14
CARBS: 34
NET CARBS: 24
FIBER: 10
PROTEIN: 12

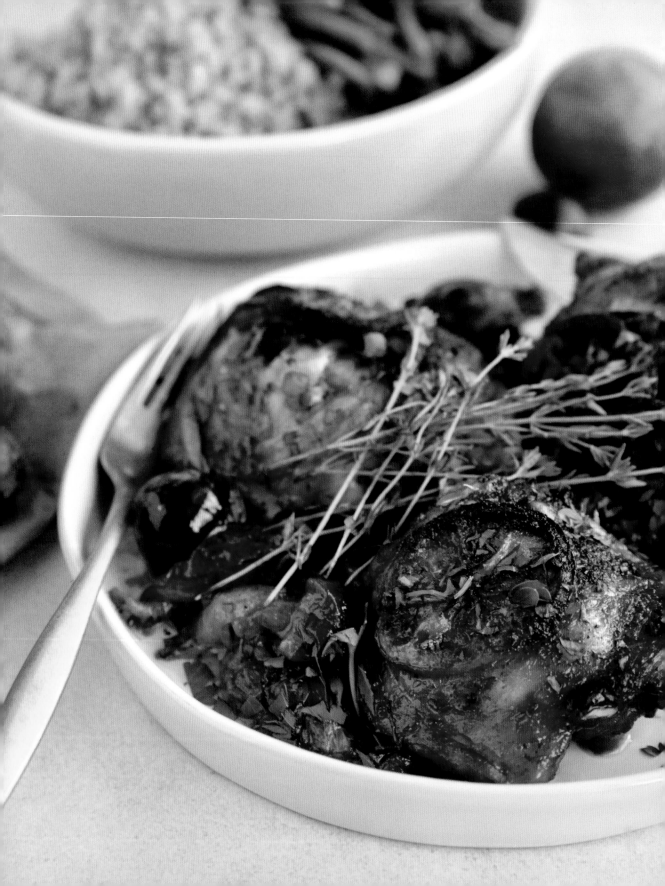

CHAPTER NINE

DINNER

Dinner doesn't have to be complicated to be good. Try these easy-to-make whole food recipes that feature several anti-inflammatory properties. You will find options like soups, salad, rice bowls, quinoa, pasta dishes, and more! Whether you are vegan or embrace animal protein, you will find an option in every recipe.

When we enjoy a meal at a restaurant, so often the greatest contributor to inflammation comes from the sauces and oils used. That's typically why most people feel inflamed or like they've retained water after eating out. The beauty of these dinner recipes is that they combine all the tasty vegetables and herbs, but they are cooked with anti-inflammatory oils such as avocado and olive oil. All the sauces are made from scratch, using ingredients such as lemon, oil, garlic, and tahini. They are not just *not inflammatory*, but they are *anti-inflammatory*, actually helping you reduce inflammation as you eat.

With a little meal planning and prep throughout your week, it is it easy to ensure the entire family is getting their immunity food fix with these nutritious dinner recipes.

Roasted Plum Chicken with Quinoa and
Green Beans, page 170

roasted sweet potatoes and tofu over kale

with spiced tahini sauce

SERVINGS: 4
PREP TIME: 10 MIN
COOK TIME: 35 MIN

VEGETARIAN
VEGAN
DAIRY-FREE
GLUTEN-FREE
GRAIN-FREE
(NON-VEGAN OPTION)

superfoods used

SWEET POTATO
TOFU
KALE
SESAME SEED
GARLIC
OLIVE OIL

nutrition info

CALORIES: 602
FAT: 32
CARBS: 54
NET CARBS: 48
FIBER: 6
PROTEIN: 25

*nutrition info for
non-vegan option*

CALORIES: 614
FAT: 30
CARBS: 53
NET CARBS: 47
FIBER: 6
PROTEIN: 35

This salad is a nutritional powerhouse with ingredients such as sweet potato, tofu, kale, and tahini (sesame seed paste). Tahini gives this recipe an excellent source of fiber, and the sweet potatoes bring vitamin A, which is essential to maintain the integrity of our mucous membranes. Sweet potatoes also break down slowly and stabilize blood sugar levels. Every bite contains vitamins and minerals to keep your immunity strong. Make a big batch of this salad and pack leftovers in your lunch for the next day!

TOFU AND SWEET POTATOES

14 ounces (400 g) extra-firm tofu
(or 1 pound (454 g) boneless,
skinless chicken breast)

2 tablespoons (30 ml) avocado oil

1 teaspoon (6 g) sea salt

½ teaspoon (3 g) black pepper

1 teaspoon (4 g) smoked paprika

3 medium (390 g) sweet potatoes,
peeled and diced

1 medium (40 g) shallot, minced

KALE

2 tablespoons (30 ml) avocado oil

2 tablespoons (30 ml) fresh lime
juice

½ teaspoon (3 g) sea salt

1 tablespoon (5 g) nutritional yeast

8 cups (168 g) chopped dinosaur
kale

TAHINI SAUCE

¼ cup (60 g) tahini

1 tablespoon (15 ml) olive oil

1 tablespoon (15 ml) raw apple
cider vinegar

1 tablespoon (15 ml) coconut
aminos

1 small (4 g) clove garlic, minced

1 teaspoon (6 g) sea salt

½ teaspoon (3 g) black pepper

GARNISH

1 tablespoon (10 g) black or white
sesame seeds

¼ cup (4 g) fresh cilantro, minced

Preheat the oven to 425°F (220°C). Line a baking sheet with parchment paper.

To make the tofu and sweet potatoes, pat dry the tofu (or chicken breast) and cut into bite-size pieces. In a large mixing bowl, add the oil, salt, pepper, and smoked paprika and whisk to combine. Add the sweet potatoes, tofu (or chicken breast), and shallot, and toss gently until coated. Arrange on the prepared baking sheet and bake in the oven for 30 to 35 minutes, tossing at the halfway mark.

Meanwhile, prepare the kale. Add the oil, lime juice, salt, and nutritional yeast to a large mixing bowl. Stir together well. Add the kale and massage into the mixture so that the kale softens and is fully coated. Set aside.

To make the tahini sauce, add all the ingredients to a blender. Blend on high speed until very creamy, scraping down the sides as needed. If it is too thick for your preference, add 1 tablespoon (15 ml) of water and blend, repeating until it is to your liking. Pour into a glass jar.

Remove the potatoes and tofu (or chicken) from the oven. Toss it with the massaged kale. Serve with the sauce, garnished with the sesame seeds and cilantro. Store any leftovers in the fridge in an airtight container for up to 5 days.

smoky black bean and butternut tacos

with pumpkin seeds

SERVINGS: 4
PREP TIME: 10 MIN
COOK TIME: 30 MIN

VEGAN
VEGETARIAN
DAIRY-FREE
GLUTEN-FREE
(NON-VEGAN OPTION)

Pepitas are a type of pumpkin seed, rich in antioxidants, iron, zinc, magnesium, manganese, and copper. Here, the butternut squash is unique but important. It is an excellent source of carotenoids, which support your immune system, and helps control blood sugar, which has a positive impact on your metabolic flexibility. The beans add protein and fiber for an overall nutritious, delicious meal on your next taco Tuesday!

superfoods used

AVOCADO OIL
BUTTERNUT SQUASH
GARLIC
TEMPEH
AVOCADO
RADISH
PUMPKIN SEED

nutrition info

CALORIES: 556
FAT: 24
CARBS: 72
NET CARBS: 48
FIBER: 24
PROTEIN: 28

*nutrition info for
non-vegan option*

CALORIES: 555
FAT: 25
CARBS: 57
NET CARBS: 36
FIBER: 21
PROTEIN: 28

TACOS

- 8 ounces (228 g) tempeh, crumbled (or 8 ounces [228 g] ground turkey)
- 8 gluten-free soft taco shells

BUTTERNUT TACO FILLING

- 2 tablespoons (30 ml) avocado oil
- 1 teaspoon (6 g) sea salt
- ½ teaspoon (3 g) black pepper
- 4 cups (820 g) cubed butternut squash
- 1 medium (40 g) shallot, minced

SMOKY BLACK BEANS

- 1 tablespoon (15 ml) avocado oil
- Zest from ½ medium (22 g) fresh lime
- 1 tablespoon (15 ml) fresh lime juice
- ½ teaspoon (3 g) sea salt
- 1 small (4 g) clove garlic, minced
- 1 teaspoon (5 g) smoked paprika
- 1 teaspoon (5) ground cumin
- 1 teaspoon (5) chili powder
- 15 ounces (425 g) cooked black beans, rinsed

GARNISH

- 1 medium (150 g) avocado, peeled, pitted, and diced
- ¼ cup (28 g) pepitas, toasted
- ½ cup (66 g) minced radish
- ¼ cup (4 g) fresh cilantro, minced

If preparing the non-vegan option, add the turkey to a large, nonstick skillet and sauté over medium-low heat until fully cooked though, breaking it up as you go, about 10 minutes. Drain and set aside.

Preheat the oven to 400°F (200°C). Line a baking sheet with parchment paper.

To make the butternut filling, add the oil, salt, and pepper to a large mixing bowl. Add the butternut and shallot and gently toss to coat. Arrange on the lined baking sheet and bake in the oven for 30 minutes, tossing at the halfway mark.

Meanwhile, prepare the smoky black beans. In a large mixing bowl, add the oil, lime zest and juice, salt, garlic, smoked paprika, cumin, and chili powder. Stir together well. Add the black beans and crumbled tempeh (or cooked turkey) and gently toss together. Heat in a sauté pan over low heat while the butternut continues to cook.

Remove the butternut from the oven and toss with the smoky black beans. Serve in grain-free soft taco shells, garnished with the avocado, pepitas, radish, and cilantro. Store any leftovers in the fridge in an airtight container for up to 5 days.

crispy miso brussels sprouts and tempeh

over quinoa with sage and almond butter sauce

SERVINGS: 4
PREP TIME: 10 MIN
PLUS SOAKING
OVERNIGHT
COOK TIME: 25 MIN

VEGETARIAN
VEGAN
DAIRY-FREE
GLUTEN-FREE
(NON-VEGAN OPTION)

superfoods used

AVOCADO OIL
BRUSSELS SPROUTS
TEMPEH
QUINOA
ALMOND
GARLIC
SAGE
HEMP SEED

nutrition info

CALORIES: 493
FAT: 26
CARBS: 55
NET CARBS: 44
FIBER: 11
PROTEIN: 25

*nutrition info for
non-vegan option*

CALORIES: 473
FAT: 24
CARBS: 41
NET CARBS: 32
FIBER: 9
PROTEIN: 26

This recipe combines the umami flavors of miso and coconut aminos with fresh sage, an herb known to fight cancer and reduce inflammation. Brussels sprouts contain biochemicals that promote detoxification, increase antioxidant activity, and reduce inflammation. The high fiber content directly effects your gut and satiety. The quinoa adds a complete plant protein that is high in fiber and phytochemicals. Its nutrition is impressive, and so are its taste and texture!

BRUSSELS SPROUTS AND TEMPEH

- 2 tablespoons (30 ml) avocado oil
- 1 teaspoon (6 g) sea salt
- ½ teaspoon (3 g) black pepper
- 1 tablespoon (17 g) light miso paste
- 2 tablespoons (30 ml) hot water
- 1 tablespoon (15 ml) coconut aminos
- 1 tablespoon (8 g) stone-ground mustard
- 12 ounces (352 g) Brussels sprouts, chopped
- 8 ounces (227 g) tempeh, crumbled (or 8 ounces [228 g] boneless, skinless chicken breast)
- 1 medium (40 g) shallot, minced

Preheat the oven to 400°F (200°C). Line a baking sheet with parchment paper.

To make the Brussels sprouts and tempeh, add the oil, salt, pepper, miso paste, hot water, coconut aminos, and mustard to a mixing bowl. Whisk together until creamy. Add the Brussels sprouts, tempeh (or chicken breast), and shallot to the bowl. Toss gently to coat. Spread in an even layer on the prepared baking sheet and bake in the oven for 20 minutes, tossing at the halfway mark.

To make the quinoa, rinse it well in a fine-mesh strainer, then transfer to a saucepan and add the boiling water over low heat. Let the quinoa soak in the boiling water for about 10 minutes, or until it has soaked up all the water.

To make the sauce, add all the ingredients to a blender and blend on high speed until very creamy, scraping down the sides as needed. If it is too thick for your preference, add 1 tablespoon (15 ml) of water and blend again, repeating until it is to your liking. Pour into a glass jar until ready to serve.

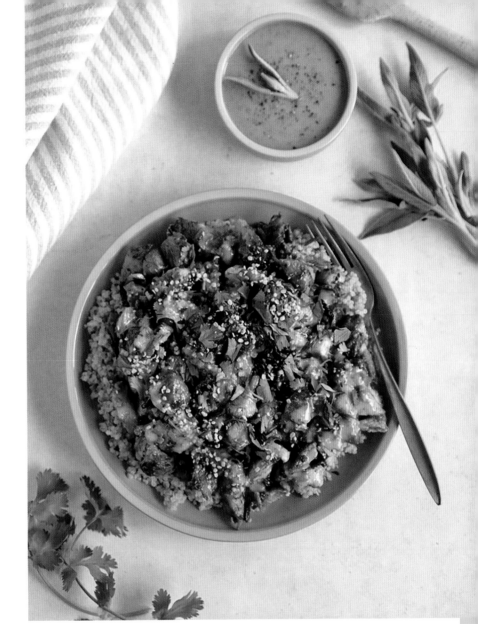

QUINOA

- 1 cup (200 g) quinoa (soaked overnight in cold water)
- 1¼ cups (300 ml) boiling water

ALMOND BUTTER SAUCE

- ¼ cup (60 g) raw almond butter
- 1 tablespoon (15 ml) olive oil
- 1 tablespoon (15 ml) coconut aminos
- 1 small (4 g) clove garlic, minced
- 1 teaspoon (6 g) sea salt
- ½ teaspoon (3 g) black pepper
- 3 fresh sage leaves, minced

GARNISH

- 1 tablespoon (10 g) hemp seeds
- ¼ cup (4 g) fresh cilantro, minced

Remove the Brussels sprouts and tempeh (or chicken) from the oven. Serve over the quinoa with the sauce and garnish with the hemp seeds and cilantro. Store any leftovers in the fridge in an airtight container for up to 5 days.

spiced lentils

with tomatoes and red potatoes

SERVINGS: 4
PREP TIME: 10 MIN
COOK TIME: 30 MIN

VEGETARIAN
VEGAN
DAIRY-FREE
GLUTEN-FREE
GRAIN-FREE

superfoods used

AVOCADO OIL
GARLIC
OREGANO
RED POTATO
ONION
TOMATO
SESAME SEED
LENTIL

nutrition info

CALORIES: 465
FAT: 20
CARBS: 52
NET CARBS: 45
FIBER: 7
PROTEIN: 15

On their own, lentils are an incomplete protein, so pair this with some brown rice to ensure you are getting the benefits of a complete nine essential amino acid meal.

RED POTATOES

- 2 tablespoons (30 g) avocado oil
- 2 small (8 g) cloves garlic, minced
- 1 teaspoon (6 g) sea salt
- ½ teaspoon (3 g) black pepper
- 1 tablespoon (3 g) fresh oregano
- 2 large (600 g) red potatoes, chopped into bite-size pieces

TOMATOES

- 1 tablespoon (15 g) avocado oil
- 1 medium (150 g) yellow onion, diced
- 1 small (4 g) clove garlic, minced
- 1 can (14.5 ounces, or 411 g) diced tomatoes
- 1 teaspoon (6 g) sea salt
- ½ teaspoon (3 g) black pepper
- 1 teaspoon (4 g) smoked paprika
- ¼ cup (60 g) tahini

LENTILS

- 1 cup (200 g) dry green lentils
- 3 cups (720 ml) water

Preheat the oven to 425°F (220°C). Line a baking sheet with parchment paper.

To make the potatoes, add the oil, garlic, salt, pepper, and oregano to a mixing bowl and whisk together until creamy. Add the red potatoes and gently toss until coated.

Spread in an even layer on the prepared baking sheet. Bake in the oven for 30 minutes, tossing at the halfway mark.

To make the tomatoes, add the oil to a sauté pan over medium-low heat. Add the onion and garlic and sauté until soft, about 5 minutes. Add the tomatoes, salt, pepper, smoked paprika, and tahini. Stir well. Decrease the heat to a simmer and cook, loosely covered, for 20 minutes, stirring often.

Meanwhile, prepare the lentils. Add the lentils and water to a medium-size pot and bring to a boil. Once boiling, decrease the heat to a simmer and cover with a lid. Simmer for 15 to 20 minutes, or until the lentils are soft. Remove from the heat and drain any excess water. Add to the pan of simmering tomatoes and stir together well.

Remove the red potatoes from the oven. Serve over the spiced lentils and tomatoes, and garnish with fresh oregano (1 tablespoon [3 g]) and parsley (¼ cup [15g]). Store any leftovers in the fridge in an airtight container for up to 5 days.

thai-spiced coconut lentil soup

SERVINGS: 4
PREP TIME: 10 MIN
COOK TIME: 30 MIN

VEGETARIAN
VEGAN
DAIRY-FREE
GLUTEN-FREE
GRAIN-FREE

This dish is best served with a side of fluffy brown rice or quinoa because lentils require a whole grain to be considered a complete protein. But the best part is the addition of turmeric, cinnamon, and ginger in this recipe! Turmeric and ginger combined have a strong anti-inflammatory presence. The active constituents in cinnamon also carry an anti-inflammatory effect, but it's the effect of cinnamon on blood sugar that's truly excellent. Prepare a batch of rice while your lentil soup is cooking (or reheat leftovers) and serve with this fragrant and delicious dish!

superfoods used

AVOCADO OIL
ONION
TURMERIC
CINNAMON
GINGER
KALE
LENTIL

nutrition info

CALORIES: 505
FAT: 25
CARBS: 47
NET CARBS: 37
FIBER: 10
PROTEIN: 20

SOUP

- 2 tablespoons (30 g) avocado oil
- 1 medium (150 g) yellow onion, minced
- 4 small (16 g) cloves garlic, minced
- 1 teaspoon (6 g) sea salt
- ½ teaspoon (3 g) black pepper
- 1 tablespoon (15 g) red curry paste
- 1 teaspoon (2 g) ground turmeric
- 1 teaspoon (3 g) dried red pepper flakes
- ½ teaspoon (3 g) ground cinnamon
- Pinch of ground nutmeg
- 1 teaspoon (2 g) peeled and minced fresh ginger
- 1½ cups (300 g) dry green or yellow lentils
- 1 can (14 ounces, or 400 ml) full-fat coconut milk
- 4 cups (960 ml) vegetable stock
- 2 tablespoons (30 ml) coconut aminos
- 4 cups (85 g) chopped dinosaur kale

GARNISH

- ¼ cup (4 g) fresh cilantro, minced
- 1 medium (15 g) scallion, minced

To make the soup, add the oil to a large pot over medium-low heat. Add the onion, garlic, salt, pepper, curry paste, turmeric, red pepper flakes, cinnamon, nutmeg, and ginger. Stir well. Sauté until the onions and garlic are soft and a bit golden, 5 to 7 minutes.

Add the lentils, coconut milk, vegetable stock, and coconut aminos. Stir well. Simmer for 12 to 15 minutes, or until the lentils are soft. Add the kale and stir until wilted. Turn off the heat.

Serve garnished with the cilantro and scallion. Store any leftovers in the fridge in an airtight container for up to 5 days.

carrot and persimmon salad

with pomegranate arils, pistachios, and mint

SERVINGS: 6
PREP TIME: 10 MIN
PLUS SOAKING
OVERNIGHT
COOK TIME: 35 MIN

VEGETARIAN
VEGAN
DAIRY-FREE
GLUTEN-FREE

superfoods used

QUINOA
CARROT
AVOCADO OIL
BASIL
PERSIMMON
PISTACHIO
POMEGRANATE ARIL
PEPPERMINT
KALE
SUNFLOWER SEED
GARLIC

nutrition info

CALORIES: 499
FAT: 23
CARBS: 63
NET CARBS: 52
FIBER: 11
PROTEIN: 11

This salad is stunning, and its bright colors means it's full of antioxidants, vitamins, and minerals. Carrots are an excellent source of carotenoids and antioxidant activity, but don't peel the carrot! About 50 percent of those benefits lie in the skin. We boost that carotenoid content with persimmon. The red pomegranate arils add delicious flavor, antioxidants, and prebiotics for the gut! Serve this at a holiday gathering alongside protein, such as chicken breast, salmon fillet, tofu, or tempeh.

QUINOA

- 1 cup (200 g) quinoa (soaked overnight in cold water)
- 1¼ cups (300 ml) boiling water

CARROTS

- 2 tablespoons (30 ml) avocado oil
- 1 teaspoon (6 g) sea salt
- ½ teaspoon (3 g) black pepper
- 1 teaspoon (4 g) smoked paprika
- 1½ teaspoons (2 g) dried basil
- 6 medium (480 g) carrots, ends trimmed and chopped in 1" rounds
- 1 medium (40 g) shallot, minced

MIXED GREENS

- 2 tablespoons (30 ml) avocado oil
- 2 tablespoons (30 ml) fresh lime juice
- ½ teaspoon (3 g) sea salt
- ¼ teaspoon (2 g) black pepper
- 1 medium (168 g) fresh persimmon, diced
- ¼ cup (28 g) raw pistachios
- ½ cup (72 g) pomegranate arils
- ¼ cup (4 g) fresh mint, minced
- 8 cups (360 g) mixed greens, such as kale, spinach, arugula, or radicchio

SUNFLOWER SEED SAUCE

- ¼ cup (34 g) shelled sunflower seeds
- 2 tablespoons (30 ml) olive oil
- 1 tablespoon (15 ml) raw apple cider vinegar
- 1 tablespoon (15 ml) fresh lime juice
- 1 tablespoon (15 ml) water
- 1 small (4 g) clove garlic, minced
- 1 teaspoon (6 g) sea salt
- ½ teaspoon (3 g) black pepper

Preheat the oven to 400°F (200°C). Line a baking sheet with parchment paper.

To make the quinoa, rinse the soaked quinoa well in a fine-mesh strainer, then transfer to a saucepan and add the boiling water over low heat. Let the quinoa soak in the boiling water for about 10 minutes, or until it has soaked up all the water.

To make the carrots, add the oil, salt, pepper, smoked paprika, and basil to a large mixing bowl and whisk to blend. Add the carrots and shallot and toss until coated. Arrange on the prepared baking sheet and bake in the oven for 25 to 30 minutes, tossing at the halfway mark.

Meanwhile, prepare the mixed greens. In a large mixing bowl, add the oil, lime juice, salt, and pepper and whisk to blend. Add the persimmon, pistachios, pomegranate arils, and mint. Stir together well. Add the greens and quinoa. Gently toss until fully coated, allowing the warm quinoa to wilt the greens. Set aside.

To make the sauce, add all the ingredients to a blender. Blend on high speed until very creamy, scraping down the sides as needed. If it is too thick for your preference, add 1 tablespoon (15 ml) of water and blend again, repeating until it is to your liking.

Remove the carrots from the oven. Toss them with the greens and quinoa, and serve with the sauce. Store any leftovers in the fridge in an airtight container for up to 5 days.

golden coconut tofu bowls

with bok choy and broccoli

SERVINGS: 4
PREP TIME: 10 MIN
PLUS SOAKING
OVERNIGHT
COOK TIME: 35 MIN

VEGAN
VEGETARIAN
DAIRY-FREE
GLUTEN-FREE
(NON-VEGAN OPTION)

superfoods used

QUINOA
TOFU
AVOCADO OIL
ONION
GARLIC
TURMERIC
GINGER
BOK CHOY
BROCCOLI

nutrition info

CALORIES: 518
FAT: 27
CARBS: 44
NET CARBS: 37
FIBER: 7
PROTEIN: 22

*nutrition info for
non-vegan option*

CALORIES: 502
FAT: 24
CARBS: 42
NET CARBS: 36
FIBER: 6
PROTEIN: 28

This recipe creates a crispy tofu (or perfectly baked shrimp) with the combination of avocado oil, arrowroot powder, and seasonings. Use this as a base and add spices you like (such as smoked paprika, cumin, or curry powder) in any recipe calling for extra-firm tofu. Bok choy is a perfect addition to this bowl. It has more than seventy antioxidants, vitamin C, and vitamin A, and it's a great source of omega-3 fatty acids, which help reduce inflammation.

QUINOA

- 1 cup (200 g) quinoa (soaked overnight in cold water)
- 1¼ cups (300 ml) boiling water

TOFU

- 14 ounces (400 g) extra-firm tofu (or 1 pound [454 g] medium-size wild-caught, tail-on shrimp)
- 1 tablespoon (15 ml) avocado oil
- 1 teaspoon (6 g) sea salt
- ½ teaspoon (3 g) black pepper
- 1 tablespoon (10 g) arrowroot powder
- 2 tablespoons (10 g) nutritional yeast

GOLDEN COCONUT BROTH

- 1 tablespoon (15 g) avocado oil
- ½ medium (75 g) yellow onion, minced
- 4 small (16 g) cloves garlic, minced
- 1 teaspoon (6 g) sea salt
- ½ teaspoon (3 g) black pepper
- 1 tablespoon (8 g) ground turmeric
- 1 teaspoon (3 g) dried red pepper flakes
- 1 teaspoon (2 g) peeled and minced fresh ginger
- 1 can (14 ounces, or 400 ml) full-fat coconut milk
- 2 tablespoons (30 ml) coconut aminos
- Zest from ½ medium (11 g) fresh lime
- 1 tablespoon (15 ml) fresh lime juice
- 4½ ounces (140 g) bok choy, ends trimmed and chopped
- 4 cups (184 g) broccoli florets, chopped

GARNISH

- ¼ cup (4 g) fresh cilantro, minced
- 1 medium (15 g) scallion, minced

Preheat the oven to 400°F (200°C). Line a baking sheet with parchment paper.

To make the quinoa, rinse the soaked quinoa well using a fine-mesh strainer, then transfer to a saucepan and add the boiling water over low heat. Let the quinoa soak in the boiling water for about 10 minutes, or until it has soaked up all the water.

To make the tofu, pat it dry and chop it into bite-size pieces. Add the oil, salt, pepper, arrowroot powder, and nutritional yeast to a large mixing bowl. Gently toss the tofu (or shrimp) in the mixture until coated. Arrange on the prepared baking sheet and bake in the oven for 15 minutes.

Meanwhile, prepare the broth. Add the avocado oil to a medium-size pot over medium-low heat. Add the onion, garlic, salt, pepper, turmeric, red pepper flakes, and ginger. Stir well. Sauté until the onions and garlic are soft and a bit golden, 5 to 7 minutes.

Add the coconut milk, coconut aminos, and lime zest and juice. Stir well. Simmer for about 10 minutes. Add the bok choy and broccoli and continue to simmer for 8 to 10 minutes, or until the vegetables are soft.

Remove the tofu (or shrimp) from the oven. Add it to the golden coconut broth. Serve with the quinoa and garnish with the cilantro and scallion. Store any leftovers in the fridge in an airtight container for up to 5 days.

sautéed cauliflower and green beans

with chickpeas and tahini

SERVINGS: 4
PREP TIME: 10 MIN
COOK TIME: 35 MIN

VEGAN
VEGETARIAN
DAIRY-FREE
GLUTEN-FREE
GRAIN-FREE

superfoods used

AVOCADO OIL
GARLIC
CHICKPEA
THYME
SESAME SEED
PUMPKIN SEED

nutrition info

CALORIES: 515
FAT: 23
CARBS: 59
NET CARBS: 46
FIBER: 13
PROTEIN: 23

This recipe is full of nutrients and has the most satisfying flavor. Thyme is an excellent add here because of its strong antioxidant and antibacterial properties. The active component thymol also has a strong antioxidant effect.

CAULIFLOWER AND GREEN BEANS

- 1 tablespoon (15 ml) avocado oil
- 1 medium (40 g) shallot, minced
- 2 small (8 g) cloves garlic, minced
- 1 teaspoon (6 g) sea salt
- ½ teaspoon (3 g) black pepper
- 4 cups (400 g) cauliflower florets
- 1 pound (454 g) fresh green beans, ends trimmed and chopped
- 15 ounces (425 g) cooked chickpeas, rinsed
- 2 teaspoons (2 g) fresh thyme

TAHINI DRESSING

- ¼ cup (60 g) tahini
- 1 tablespoon (15 ml) olive oil
- 1 tablespoon (15 ml) raw apple cider vinegar
- 1 tablespoon (15 ml) fresh lemon juice
- 1 small (4 g) clove garlic, minced
- 1 teaspoon (6 g) sea salt
- ½ teaspoon (3 g) black pepper
- 1 tablespoon (5 g) nutritional yeast

GARNISH

- ¼ cup (28 g) pumpkin seeds
- ¼ cup (4 g) fresh parsley, minced

To make the cauliflower and green beans, add the oil to a large skillet over medium-low heat. Add the shallot, garlic, salt, and pepper. Sauté until the shallot and garlic are soft and a bit golden, about 5 minutes. Add the cauliflower and green beans. Continue to sauté over low heat, covered, until soft, 8 to 10 minutes.

While the cauliflower and green beans are cooking, prepare the tahini dressing. Add all the ingredients to a blender. Blend on high speed until very creamy, scraping down the sides of the blender as needed.

When the cauliflower and green beans are soft, add the chickpeas and thyme, stir together well, and remove from the heat.

Serve with the tahini dressing, pumpkin seeds, and parsley. Store any leftovers in the fridge in an airtight container for up to 5 days.

seared salmon

with avocado mash over herbed brown rice

The avocado mash takes your salmon to the next level, and you're compounding the omega-3 fatty acid intake with this combination. It's wonderful with a side of steamed bok choy, spinach, or broccoli; for extra protein and fiber, stir in ½ cup (170 g) each of chickpeas and edamame.

BROWN RICE

- 1 cup (200 g) brown rice
- 2 cups (480 ml) water
- ¼ cup (4 g) fresh cilantro, minced
- 1 medium (15 g) scallion, minced
- Zest from ½ medium (22 g) fresh lime

SALMON

- 1 tablespoon (15 g) avocado oil
- 1 pound (454 g) wild-caught salmon fillets (or 1 pound [454 g] extra-firm tofu, sliced)
- 1 teaspoon (6 g) sea salt
- ½ teaspoon (3 g) black pepper

AVOCADO MASH

- 2 medium (300 g) avocados, peeled, pitted, and chopped
- 1 teaspoon (6 g) sea salt
- ½ teaspoon (3 g) black pepper
- ¼ cup (4 g) fresh cilantro, minced
- Zest from ½ medium (11 g) fresh lime
- 2 tablespoons (30 ml) fresh lime juice

GARNISH

- 2 tablespoons (20 g) hemp seeds

To make the rice, rinse it well in a fine-mesh strainer. Add it and water to a large pot on the stove. Cover and bring to a boil. Once boiling, decrease the heat to a simmer and cook until soft and fluffy, 40 to 45 minutes. When it is done, remove from the heat and stir in the cilantro, scallion, and zest.

While the rice is cooking, make the salmon (or tofu). Add the oil to a large skillet over medium-high heat. Season the salmon (or tofu) with salt and pepper. Place the salmon fillets (or tofu) in the skillet, skin-side down, not moving them once in the skillet. Sear for 3 to 4 minutes per side, or until the flesh is opaque (or golden, if using tofu). Turn off the heat.

To make the mash, add the avocado to a bowl and gently mash with a potato masher or the back of a fork. Season with the salt, pepper, cilantro, and lime zest and juice. Gently mix together. Set aside.

Serve the salmon (or tofu) over the herbed brown rice, garnishing with the mashed avocado and hemp seeds. Store any leftovers in the fridge in an airtight container for up to 2 days.

SERVINGS: 4
PREP TIME: 10 MIN
COOK TIME: 50 MIN

DAIRY-FREE
GLUTEN-FREE
(VEGAN OPTION)

superfoods used

LIME
AVOCADO OIL
AVOCADO
HEMP SEED
SALMON

nutrition info

CALORIES: 546
FAT: 27
CARBS: 39
NET CARBS: 32
FIBER: 7
PROTEIN: 31

nutrition info for vegan option

CALORIES: 500
FAT: 25
CARBS: 41
NET CARBS: 34
FIBER: 7
PROTEIN: 23

roasted asparagus salad

with tempeh, white beans, and radish in lemon zest vinaigrette with brazil nut crumble

SERVINGS: 4
PREP TIME: 15 MIN
COOK TIME: 15 MIN

VEGAN
VEGETARIAN
DAIRY-FREE
GLUTEN-FREE
(NON-VEGAN OPTION)

superfoods used

AVOCADO OIL
TEMPEH
KALE
RADISH
OLIVE OIL
BRAZIL NUT
GARLIC
ASPARAGUS

nutrition info

CALORIES: 502
FAT: 22
CARBS: 63
NET CARBS: 41
FIBER: 22
PROTEIN: 32

nutrition info for non-vegan option

CALORIES: 542
FAT: 26
CARBS: 42
NET CARBS: 25
FIBER: 17
PROTEIN: 38

Look for Brazil nuts with their skin on, as the skin contains a significant portion of its polyphenols. Asparagus is an excellent source of inulin, a prebiotic to support gut health. It also contains quercetin, a key polyphenol with anti-inflammatory and antioxidant activity that has an impact on viral replication. The beans bring protein and fiber to this recipe. Whether you choose to make this vegan or non-vegan, you are looking at a well-rounded macros meal!

ASPARAGUS

- 12 ounces (340 g) tempeh, chopped into bite-size pieces (or 1 pound [454 g] ground turkey)
- 1 tablespoon (15 ml) avocado oil
- 2 small (8 g) cloves garlic, minced
- 1 teaspoon (6 g) sea salt
- ½ teaspoon (3 g) black pepper
- 1 pound (454 g) asparagus, tough ends trimmed and chopped
- 1 medium (40 g) shallot, minced

Preheat the oven to 425°F (220°C). Line a baking sheet with parchment paper.

If preparing the non-vegan option, add the turkey to a large, nonstick skillet and sauté over medium-low heat until fully cooked though, breaking it up as you go, for about 10 minutes. Drain and set aside.

To make the asparagus, add the oil, garlic, salt, and pepper to a large mixing bowl. Add the tempeh, asparagus, and shallot and toss gently until coated. Arrange on the prepared baking sheet and bake in the oven for 15 minutes, tossing at the halfway mark.

Meanwhile, prepare the vinaigrette. In a large mixing bowl, add the oil, vinegar, lemon zest and juice, salt, pepper, and parsley. Stir together well.

To make the salad, add the baby kale, white beans, and radish to the bowl with the vinaigrette. Toss until fully coated.

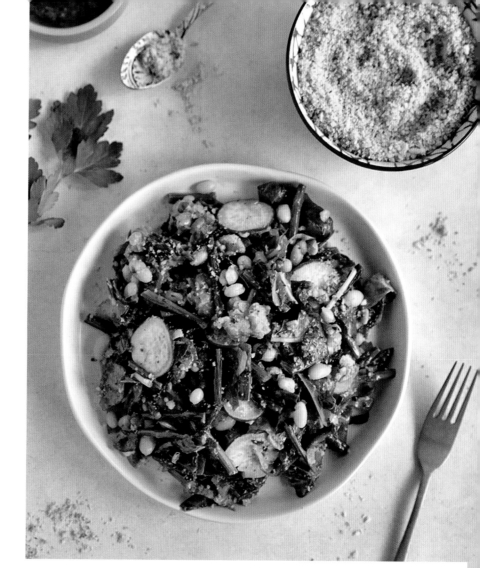

LEMON ZEST VINAIGRETTE

- 3 tablespoon (45 ml) olive oil
- 1 tablespoon (15 ml) raw apple cider vinegar
- 2 teaspoons (4 g) fresh lemon zest
- 2 tablespoon (30 ml) fresh lemon juice
- 1 teaspoon (6 g) sea salt
- ½ teaspoon (3 g) black pepper
- ¼ cup (4 g) fresh parsley, minced

SALAD

- 8 cups (340 g) baby kale
- 15 ounces (425 g) cooked white beans, rinsed
- ¾ cup (100 g) radishes, ends trimmed and sliced

BRAZIL NUT CRUMBLE

- ¼ cup (28 g) Brazil nuts, chopped
- 1 small (4 g) clove garlic, minced
- 1 tablespoon (5 g) nutritional yeast
- 1 teaspoon (6 g) sea salt

When the asparagus is done, remove it from the oven and add it to the salad. If preparing the non-vegan option, add the cooked turkey.

To make the Brazil nut crumble, add the nuts, garlic, nutritional yeast, and salt to a food processor. Pulse until it is coarse and crumbly, scraping down the sides of the bowl as needed.

Serve the salad garnished with the crumble. Store any leftovers in the fridge for up to 5 days.

roasted cherry and fennel quinoa salad

with pistachios and orange-almond dressing

SERVINGS: 4
PREP TIME: 10 MIN
PLUS SOAKING
OVERNIGHT
COOK TIME: 25 MIN

VEGETARIAN
VEGAN
DAIRY-FREE
GLUTEN-FREE

superfoods used

AVOCADO OIL
CHERRY
FENNEL
QUINOA
ALMOND
ORANGE
PISTACHIO

nutrition info

CALORIES: 433
FAT: 23
CARBS: 47
NET CARBS: 37
FIBER: 10
PROTEIN: 13

Cherries are an outstanding, nutrient-dense food with an abundance of polyphenols, fiber, carotenoids, and vitamin C. They also can help increase good bacteria in the gut. You can use frozen cherries in this dish if you cannot source fresh. Simply defrost them in a bowl on the counter before you slice and roast with the fennel and shallot. To increase the protein in this recipe, serve with a side of boneless, skinless chicken breast, tempeh, or chickpeas.

CHERRIES AND FENNEL

- 1½ tablespoons (25 ml) avocado oil
- 1 teaspoon (6 g) sea salt
- ½ teaspoon (3 g) black pepper
- 1½ cups (150 g) cherries, pitted and halved
- 12 ounces (360 g) fennel bulb, ends trimmed and thinly sliced
- 1 medium (40 g) shallot, minced

QUINOA

- 1 cup (200 g) quinoa (soaked overnight in cold water)
- 1¼ cups (300 ml) boiling water

Preheat the oven to 425°F (220°C). Line a baking sheet with parchment paper.

To make the cherries and fennel, add the oil, salt, and pepper to a mixing bowl. Stir to combine. Add the cherries, fennel, and shallot to the bowl. Gently toss until everything is coated. Spread in an even layer on the prepared baking sheet and bake in the oven for 20 minutes, tossing at the halfway mark.

To make the quinoa, rinse the quinoa very well in a fine-mesh strainer, then transfer to a saucepan and add the boiling water over low heat. Let the quinoa soak in the boiling water for about 10 minutes, or until it has soaked up all the water.

To make the dressing, add all the ingredients to a small bowl and whisk until very creamy. If it is too thick for your preference, add 1 tablespoon (15 ml) of water and whisk again, repeating until it is to your liking. Pour into a glass jar until ready to serve.

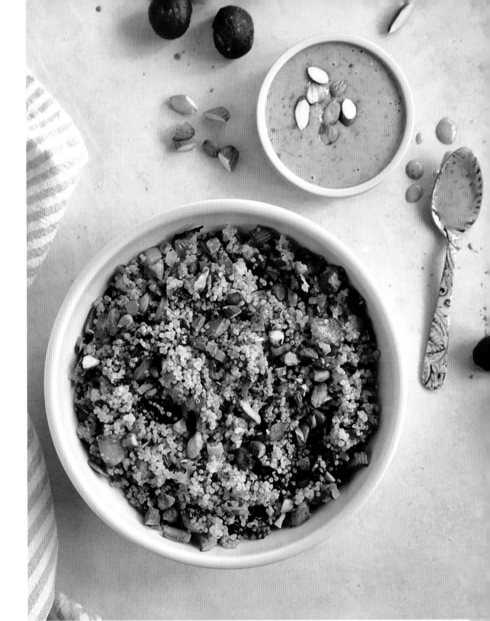

ALMOND-ORANGE DRESSING

- ¼ cup (60 g) raw almond butter
- 1 tablespoon (15 ml) olive oil
- 1 teaspoon (2 g) fresh orange zest
- 2 tablespoons (30 ml) fresh orange juice
- 1 tablespoon (15 ml) raw apple cider vinegar
- 1 teaspoon (6 g) sea salt
- ½ teaspoon (3 g) black pepper

GARNISH

- ¼ cup (31 g) shelled pistachios
- 1 medium (15 g) scallion, minced

Remove the cherries and fennel from the oven. Toss with the quinoa. Serve with the dressing, garnished with the pistachios and scallion. Store any leftovers in the fridge in an airtight container for up to 5 days.

creamy chicken and rice soup with basil and lemon

SERVINGS: 4
PREP TIME: 10 MIN
COOK TIME: 50 MIN

DAIRY-FREE
GLUTEN-FREE
(VEGAN OPTION)

This soup is warm and comforting with a pop of flavor from fresh lemon and herbs. This is the perfect soup when you are feeling under the weather, as it is a unique twist on your traditional chicken noodle soup. The simmering combination of onion, garlic, celery, and carrots speaks to the immune system with a variety of micronutrients and phytochemicals. You can freeze it for up to 3 months and reheat on a day when you have less time to cook.

superfoods used

AVOCADO OIL
ONION
GARLIC
CELERY
CARROT
LEMON
BASIL

nutrition info

CALORIES: 450
FAT: 15
CARBS: 44
NET CARBS: 39
FIBER: 5
PROTEIN: 33

nutrition info for vegan option

CALORIES: 455
FAT: 19
CARBS: 45
NET CARBS: 40
FIBER: 5
PROTEIN: 25

WILD RICE

- 1 cup (200 g) wild rice
- 6 cups (1440 ml) water

CHICKEN

- 1 tablespoon (15 g) avocado oil
- 1 pound (454 g) boneless, skinless chicken breast, chopped into bite-size pieces (or 1 pound [454 g] extra-firm tofu, cubed)
- 1 teaspoon (6 g) sea salt

To make the rice, rinse the rice well in a fine-mesh strainer. Add it with the water to a large pot on the stove. Cover and bring to a boil. Once boiling, decrease the heat to a simmer and cook until soft and fluffy, 40 to 45 minutes.

While the rice is cooking, prepare the chicken (or tofu). Add the oil to a large pot over medium-low heat. Season the chicken (or tofu) with salt and sauté until cooked through and slightly golden, about 10 minutes. When done, remove from the pot and set aside.

To make the soup, add the onion, garlic, salt, and pepper to the same pot. Sauté until the onions and garlic are soft and a bit golden, 5 to 7 minutes. Add the celery and carrot. Continue to sauté until soft, about 5 minutes. Add the coconut milk, broth, and bay leaves. Stir well. Simmer for about 10 minutes.

Add the nutritional yeast and stir well. Stir in the cooked chicken (or tofu). Add the arrowroot powder and stir well. This will help the soup thicken. Add the lemon zest and juice. Discard the bay leaves. Stir well.

When the rice is done, remove from the heat. Add the rice to the soup and stir well. Serve garnished with the parsley, basil, and scallion. Store any leftovers in the fridge in an airtight container for up to 3 days.

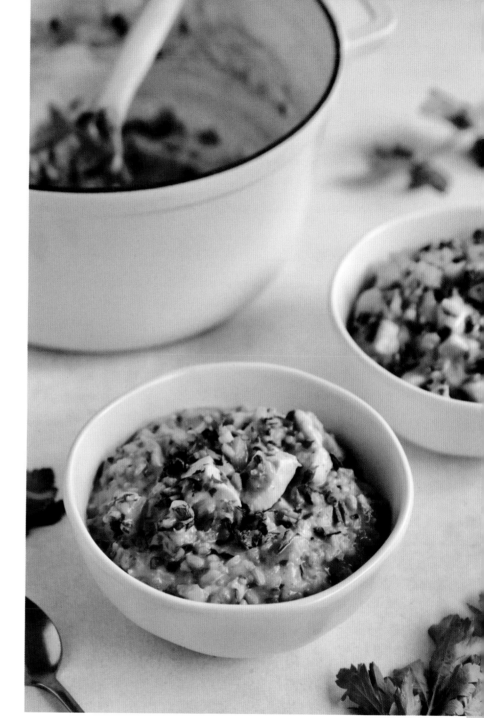

SOUP

- 1 medium (150 g) yellow onion, minced
- 4 small (16 g) cloves garlic, minced
- 1 teaspoon (6 g) sea salt
- ½ teaspoon (3 g) black pepper
- 1 cup (100 g) chopped celery
- 1 cup (150 g) chopped carrots
- 1 can (14 ounces, or 400 ml) full-fat coconut milk
- 3 cups (720 ml) chicken or vegetable stock
- 2 bay leaves
- 2 tablespoons (10 g) nutritional yeast
- 1 tablespoon (10 g) arrowroot powder
- Zest from ½ medium (13 g) fresh lemon
- 1 tablespoon (15 ml) fresh lemon juice

GARNISH

- ¼ cup (4 g) fresh parsley, minced
- 2 tablespoons (2 g) fresh basil, minced
- 1 medium (15 g) scallion, minced

moroccan-spiced carrot and parsnip salad

with lemon-roasted cod

SERVINGS: 4
PREP TIME: 15 MIN
COOK TIME: 15 MIN

DAIRY-FREE
GLUTEN-FREE
(VEGAN OPTION)

superfoods used

CARROT
PARSNIP
CINNAMON
LEMON

nutrition info

CALORIES: 411
FAT: 20
CARBS: 36
NET CARBS: 27
FIBER: 9
PROTEIN: 24

nutrition info for
vegan option

CALORIES: 448
FAT: 24
CARBS: 57
NET CARBS: 44
FIBER: 13
PROTEIN: 20

Parsnips are excellent for gut health and contain fiber, potassium, and vitamin C. They boost immunity and have natural antifungal properties. While they are similar to carrots, what differentiates them is a key active ingredient, furanocoumarin, which possesses anticancer properties. Carrots have a detox superpower with the availability of the fiber, pectin. The variety of colors gives us synergistic antioxidant capacity. Look for parsnips during the autumn season, and be sure to include them in your meals at that time of year!

SALAD

- 4 medium (260 g) carrots, ends trimmed and peeled
- 5 medium (400 g) parsnips, ends trimmed and peeled
- 1 medium (40 g) shallot, minced
- 2 tablespoons (30 ml) avocado oil
- 2 tablespoons (30 ml) fresh lemon juice
- 1 teaspoon (6 g) sea salt
- ½ teaspoon (3 g) black pepper
- 1 teaspoon (5 g) smoked paprika
- 1 teaspoon (5) ground cumin
- 1 teaspoon (3 g) ground cinnamon
- Pinch of ground nutmeg

Preheat the oven to 400°F (200°C). Line a baking sheet with parchment paper.

To make the salad, using the shredding blade on a food processor, shred the carrots and parsnips. Alternatively, you can shred them using a box grater. Set aside.

In a large mixing bowl, add the shallot, oil, lemon juice, salt, pepper, smoked paprika, cumin, cinnamon, and nutmeg. Whisk well. Stir in the minced mint, parsley, and cilantro. Gently toss the carrots and parsnips in the oil mixture until they are coated. Stir in the shallot, almonds, and raisins.

To prepare the cod (or tempeh), add the oil, lemon juice, salt, and pepper to a bowl.

Arrange the cod (or tempeh) on the prepared baking sheet and brush the oil mixture over each piece. Bake in the oven for 15 minutes.

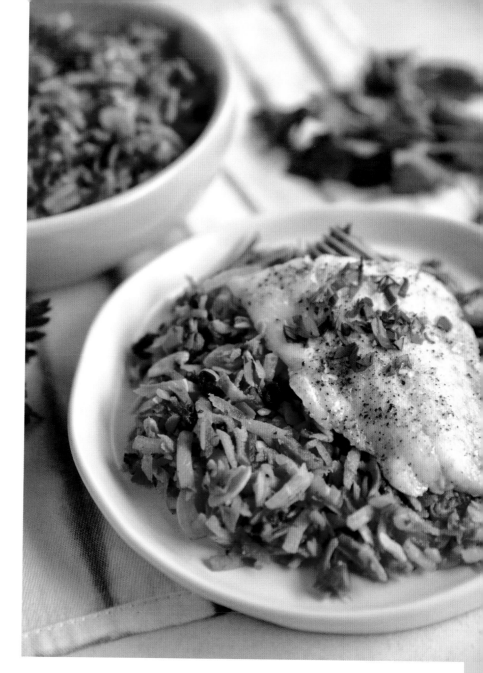

- 2 tablespoons (2 g) fresh mint, minced
- 2 tablespoons (2 g) fresh parsley, minced
- 2 tablespoons (2 g) fresh cilantro, minced
- ¼ cup (28 g) sliced almonds
- ¼ cup (40 g) raisins

COD

- 1 pound (454 g) cod fillets (or ¾ pound [342 g] tempeh, sliced into 4 pieces)
- 2 tablespoons (30 ml) avocado oil
- 1 tablespoon (15 ml) fresh lemon juice
- ½ teaspoon (3 g) sea salt
- ¼ teaspoon (2 g) black pepper
- 2 tablespoons (2 g) fresh parsley, minced

Remove the cod (or tempeh) from the oven and garnish with the parsley. Serve with the carrot and parsnip salad. Store any leftovers in the fridge in an airtight container for up to 2 days.

lemony shrimp chickpea pasta

with spinach and walnuts

SERVINGS: 4
PREP TIME: 15 MIN
COOK TIME: 20 MIN

DAIRY-FREE
GLUTEN-FREE
(VEGAN OPTION)

superfoods used

**AVOCADO OIL
LEMON
CHICKPEA
RED ONION
WALNUT**

nutrition info

**CALORIES: 491
FAT: 22
CARBS: 43
NET CARBS: 35
FIBER: 8
PROTEIN: 37**

*nutrition info for
vegan option*

**CALORIES: 396
FAT: 22
CARBS: 42
NET CARBS: 34
FIBER: 8
PROTEIN: 15**

This recipe is simple yet nutritious. Chickpea pasta is excellent as a pasta alternative because it's a high-protein, gluten-free option. It has become more available in many grocery stores (opt for varieties with only chickpeas in the ingredients). Chickpeas also provide the gut with butyrate, a key SCFA that feeds the gut microbiome. Red onions are high in anthocyanins—given that they are purple on the outside—and this speaks to the added antioxidant content.

CHICKPEA PASTA

- 8 ounces (228 g) chickpea pasta

SHRIMP

- 1 pound (454 g) shrimp, deveined (omit for vegan option)
- 2 tablespoons (30 ml) avocado oil
- 1 tablespoon (15 ml) fresh lemon juice
- ½ teaspoon (3 g) sea salt
- ¼ teaspoon (2 g) black pepper

To make the pasta, bring a large pot of water to a boil. When boiling, add the chickpea pasta and cook according to the package instructions (5 to 10 minutes). When it reaches your desired tenderness, remove from the heat and drain in a colander, reserving 1/4 cup (60 ml) of the pasta water.

To make the shrimp (if using), gently toss the shrimp in a mixing bowl with the oil, lemon juice, salt, and pepper. Place a large skillet on the stove over high heat. Sear in the hot skillet for 1 to 2 minutes per side, not moving once in the pan except to flip at the halfway mark. Remove from the heat and set aside.

To make the spinach and walnuts, in the same skillet over medium-low heat, heat the oil. Add the red onion, garlic, salt, and pepper. Sauté until soft, about 5 minutes. Add the baby spinach and stir. When wilted, turn off the heat. Add the lemon zest and juice, parsley, and walnuts. Stir in the cooked shrimp (if using).

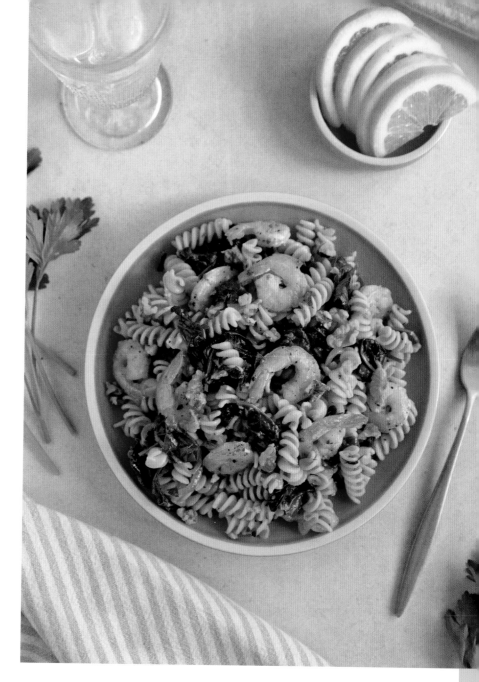

SPINACH AND WALNUTS

2 tablespoons (30 ml) avocado oil

1 medium (150 g) red onion, sliced

4 small (16 g) cloves garlic, minced

1 teaspoon (6 g) sea salt

½ teaspoon (3 g) black pepper

8 cups (240 g) baby spinach

Zest from 1 medium (13 g) fresh lemon

2 tablespoons (30 ml) fresh lemon juice

¼ cup (4 g) fresh parsley, minced

¼ cup (28 g) chopped walnuts (or ½ cup [56 g] for vegan option)

Add the skillet contents to the pasta and gently toss. You can add the reserved pasta water, 1 tablespoon (15 ml) at a time, to help coat the pasta evenly. Serve and enjoy! Store any leftovers in the fridge in an airtight container for up to 2 days.

Dinner ⸺ 161

roasted kumquat and brussels salad with cod

SERVINGS: 4
PREP TIME: 10 MIN
COOK TIME: 30 MIN

DAIRY-FREE
GLUTEN-FREE
(VEGAN OPTION)

superfoods used

AVOCADO OIL
SHALLOT
GARLIC
KUMQUAT
BRUSSELS SPROUT
MACADAMIA NUT
PEPPERMINT
LEMON
AVOCADO

nutrition info

CALORIES: 486
FAT: 27
CARBS: 37
NET CARBS: 28
FIBER: 9
PROTEIN: 21

*nutrition info for
vegan option*

CALORIES: 545
FAT: 33
CARBS: 61
NET CARBS: 48
FIBER: 13
PROTEIN: 26

Kumquats have a sweet and sour punch to their flavor. In this dish, they make a fantastic addition to the pungent, savory, and creamy flavors of Brussels sprouts, coconut aminos, and avocado.

KUMQUATS AND BRUSSELS SPROUTS

- 2 tablespoons (30 ml) avocado oil
- 2 tablespoons (30 ml) coconut aminos
- 1 medium (40 g) shallot, minced
- 2 small (8 g) cloves garlic, minced
- 1 teaspoon (6 g) sea salt
- ½ teaspoon (3 g) black pepper
- 5 ounces (150 g) fresh kumquats, halved
- 12 ounces (340 g) Brussels sprouts, chopped
- ¼ cup (28 g) chopped macadamia nuts
- 2 tablespoons (2 g) fresh mint, minced
- 2 tablespoons (2 g) fresh parsley, minced

COD

- 2 tablespoons (30 ml) avocado oil
- 1 tablespoon (15 ml) fresh lemon juice
- ½ teaspoon (3 g) sea salt
- ¼ teaspoon (2 g) black pepper
- 1½ pounds (682 g) wild-caught cod fillets (or 14 ounces [400 g] tempeh, cut into 4 pieces)

GARNISH

- 1 medium (150 g) avocado, peeled, pitted, and diced
- 2 tablespoons (2 g) fresh parsley, minced

Preheat the oven to 400°F (200°C). Line two baking sheets with parchment paper.

To make the kumquats and Brussels sprouts, in a large mixing bowl, add the oil, coconut aminos, shallot, garlic, salt, and pepper. Whisk well. Add the kumquats and Brussels sprouts and toss gently to coat. Arrange on one of the prepared baking sheets and roast in the oven for 20 minutes. At the halfway mark, toss with a spatula. When there are 5 minutes left of roasting, stir in the macadamia nuts so that they toast and turn golden, but do not burn. When done, remove from the oven and sprinkle with the mint and parsley.

To make the cod (or tempeh), add the oil, lemon juice, salt, and pepper to a bowl. Arrange the cod (or tempeh) on the second prepared baking sheet and brush the oil mixture over each piece. Bake in the oven for 15 minutes;

Remove the cod (or tempeh) from the oven. Serve with the kumquats and Brussels sprouts, garnished with the avocado and parsley. Serve and enjoy!

roasted cabbage

with chicken and mustard seed sauce

Mustard seeds are high in antioxidants and selenium. They increase strength in your bones, nails, hair, teeth, and gums, a great incentive to add it to your meals. Selenium is super important for thyroid health and thyroid hormone production. This meal combines mustard seeds with tahini and lemon to give the perfect flavor—and also brings anti-inflammatory benefits through an abundance of omega-3 fatty acids. This is a simple, great source of protein and fiber in just one meal!

SERVINGS: 4
PREP TIME: 10 MIN
COOK TIME: 35 MIN

DAIRY-FREE
GLUTEN-FREE
GRAIN-FREE
(VEGAN OPTION)

MUSTARD SEED SAUCE

- ¼ cup (60 ml) avocado oil
- ¼ cup (60 g) tahini
- 2 tablespoons (30 g) stone-ground mustard
- 2 tablespoons (30 ml) fresh lemon juice
- 2 tablespoon (30 ml) coconut aminos
- 1 teaspoon (6 g) sea salt
- ½ teaspoon (3 g) black pepper
- ½ teaspoon (3 g) garlic powder
- 1 tablespoon (6 g) mustard seeds

CABBAGE AND CHICKEN

- 1 medium (908 g) head green or purple cabbage (or ½ of each), chopped
- 1 pound (454 g) boneless, skinless chicken thighs, chopped (or 14 ounces [400 g] chopped tempeh)

GARNISH

- ¼ cup (4 g) fresh parsley, minced

Preheat the oven to 425°F (220°C). Line a baking sheet with parchment paper.

To make the sauce, add all the ingredients to a large mixing bowl. Whisk well.

To make the cabbage and chicken, add the cabbage and chicken (or tempeh) to the bowl. Gently toss until everything is coated. Arrange on the prepared baking sheet and bake in the oven for 30 minutes, tossing at the halfway mark.

Remove from the oven when the cabbage is soft and begun to brown and the chicken (or tempeh) is cooked through or has reached 165°F (74°C).

Remove the pan from the oven and garnish with the parsley. Serve and enjoy! Store any leftovers in the fridge in an airtight container for up to 3 days.

superfoods used

AVOCADO OIL
OLIVE OIL
SESAME SEED
MUSTARD SEED
LEMON
CABBAGE

nutrition info

CALORIES: 403
FAT: 29
CARBS: 20
NET CARBS: 13
FIBER: 7
PROTEIN: 25

nutrition info for vegan option

CALORIES: 442
FAT: 29
CARBS: 45
NET CARBS: 33
FIBER: 12
PROTEIN: 25

roasted root veggie soup with salmon

SERVINGS: 4
PREP TIME: 10 MIN
COOK TIME: 50 MIN

DAIRY-FREE
GLUTEN-FREE
GRAIN-FREE
(VEGAN OPTION)

superfoods used

AVOCADO OIL
ONION
GARLIC
CARROT
TURNIP
PARSNIP
SWEET POTATO
SALMON

nutrition info

CALORIES: 411
FAT: 21
CARBS: 23
NET CARBS: 17
FIBER: 6
PROTEIN: 29

*nutrition info for
vegan option*

CALORIES: 400
FAT: 17
CARBS: 52
NET CARBS: 39
FIBER: 13
PROTEIN: 13

Roasting vegetables before adding them to a soup makes their flavor pop in such a wonderful, warming way. This recipe combines all our root vegetables in one bowl. They are super nutrient dense, and that makes sense when you think about how they are grown and how nutrients are absorbed through the roots in the soil. It's important to focus on organic vegetables here. This soup is delicious served as is, or try it over a bowl of fluffy brown rice, quinoa, or cracked spelt!

VEGETABLES

- 2 tablespoons (30 ml) avocado oil
- 1 teaspoon (6 g) sea salt
- ½ teaspoon (3 g) black pepper
- 1 tablespoon (3 g) dried rosemary
- 1 medium (150 g) yellow onion, chopped
- 4 small (16 g) cloves garlic, minced
- 5 ounces (150 g) carrots, ends trimmed, peeled, and chopped
- 7 ounces (210 g) turnips, peeled and chopped
- 1 medium (130 g) sweet potato, peeled and chopped

Preheat the oven to 400°F (200°C). Line two baking sheets with parchment paper.

To make the vegetables, add the oil, salt, pepper, and rosemary to a large mixing bowl. Stir well. Add the onion, garlic, carrots, turnips, and sweet potato to the bowl. Toss together well. Arrange on one of the prepared baking sheets. Roast in the oven until everything is soft and caramelized, about 30 minutes, tossing at the halfway mark. Remove from the oven when done, leaving the oven on to cook the salmon.

To make the soup, add the roasted vegetables, stock, mustard, lemon juice, bay leaves, and nutritional yeast to a large pot over medium-low heat. Decrease the heat to a simmer and cook, uncovered, for 10 minutes. Discard the bay leaves.

While the soup is simmering, prepare the salmon (or chickpeas). Brush the oil over each fillet and season with the salt and pepper. Place on the second prepared baking sheet and bake in the oven for 10 minutes. When done, remove from the oven and shred with two forks. If preparing the vegan option, simply stir the chickpeas into the soup.

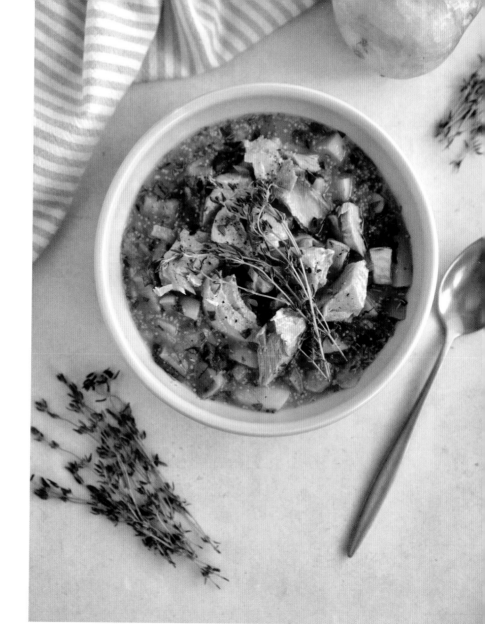

SOUP

- 3 cups (720 ml) chicken or vegetable stock
- 1 tablespoon (15 g) stone-ground mustard
- 2 tablespoons (30 ml) fresh lemon juice
- 2 bay leaves
- 2 tablespoons (10 g) nutritional yeast
- ¼ cup (4 g) fresh parsley, minced

SALMON

- 1 tablespoon (15 g) avocado oil
- 1 pound (454 g) wild-caught salmon fillets (or 2½ cups [425 g] cooked chickpeas)
- 1 teaspoon (6 g) sea salt
- ½ teaspoon (3 g) black pepper

GARNISH

- A few sprigs of fresh thyme

Serve the soup and salmon (or chickpeas) garnished with thyme. Store any leftovers in the fridge in an airtight container for up to 2 days.

sweet potato, broccoli, cherry tomato, and salmon sheet pan

SERVINGS: 4
PREP TIME: 10 MIN
COOK TIME: 35 MIN

DAIRY-FREE
GLUTEN-FREE
GRAIN-FREE
(VEGAN OPTION)

superfoods used

AVOCADO OIL
BASIL
SWEET POTATO
BROCCOLI
CHERRY TOMATO
RED ONION
SUNFLOWER SEED
SALMON

nutrition info

CALORIES: 563
FAT: 20
CARBS: 60
NET CARBS: 43
FIBER: 17
PROTEIN: 38

nutrition info for vegan option

CALORIES: 560
FAT: 22
CARBS: 61
NET CARBS: 44
FIBER: 17
PROTEIN: 30

Sheet-pan dinners are a wonderful way to create meals that are complete with protein, fiber, and healthy fats. They also make cleaning up simple! Cooking tomatoes in this recipe helps activate the lycopene, which makes it more readily absorbed, and combined with the beta-carotenes provides excellent anti-inflammatory activity. Sweet potatoes give us our resistant starch and broccoli gives it a detox boost! This recipe combines a variety of textures and flavors for ultimate satisfaction and immune-boosting benefits!

VEGETABLES AND SALMON

- 3 tablespoons (45 ml) avocado oil, divided
- 2 tablespoons (30 ml) fresh lime juice
- 1 tablespoon (15 ml) coconut aminos
- 1 teaspoon (6 g) sea salt, plus more as needed
- ½ teaspoon (3 g) black pepper, plus more as needed
- 1 teaspoon (5 g) smoked paprika
- 1 teaspoon (5 g) ground cumin
- 2 teaspoons (10 g) dried basil
- 2 small (8 g) cloves garlic, minced
- 3 medium (390 g) sweet potatoes, peeled and chopped
- 3 cups (213 g) broccoli florets
- 1½ cups (300 g) cherry tomatoes
- ½ medium (75 g) red onion, diced
- ¾ pound (342 g) wild-caught salmon fillets (or 14 ounces [400 g] extra-firm tofu, cubed)

Preheat the oven to 425°F (220°C). Line a baking sheet with parchment paper.

To make the vegetables and salmon, add 2 tablespoons (30 ml) of the oil, lime juice, coconut aminos, salt, pepper, smoked paprika, cumin, basil, and garlic to a large mixing bowl. Whisk to combine. Add the sweet potatoes, broccoli, cherry tomatoes, and red onion and toss gently to coat. Arrange on the prepared baking sheet and bake in the oven for 30 to 35 minutes, tossing at the halfway mark, which is also when you will add the salmon (or tofu).

At the halfway mark, rub the salmon with the remaining 1 tablespoon oil and sprinkle with salt and pepper. Add the salmon (or tofu) to the baking sheet, nestling it in with the vegetables.

Continue baking in the oven until the salmon (or tofu) is cooked through, the vegetables are very soft and caramelized,

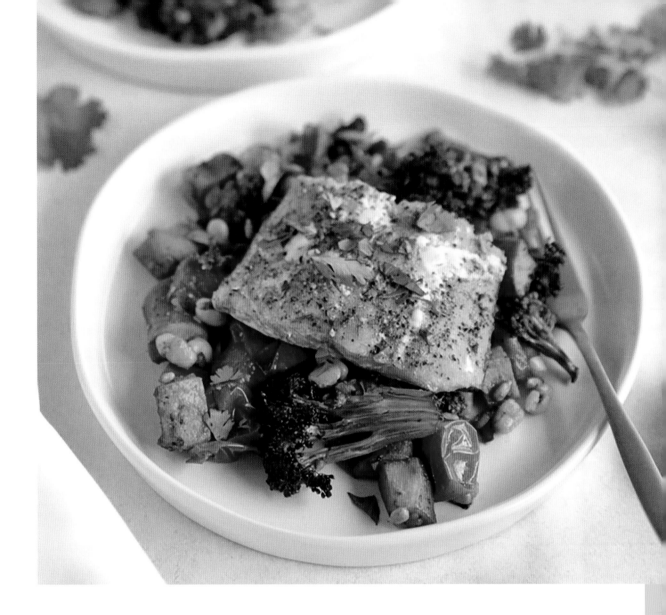

15 ounces (425 g) white navy beans, rinsed

¼ cup (28 g) sunflower seeds

GARNISH

¼ cup (4 g) fresh cilantro, minced

and the cherry tomatoes have burst open. When there are 5 minutes left of baking time, spread the white navy beans and sunflower seeds over the entire pan, gently tossing with the veggies but not moving the salmon much. This will warm the beans and lightly toast the sunflower seeds.

Remove the pan from the oven and garnish with the cilantro. Serve and enjoy! Store any leftovers in the fridge in an airtight container for up to 2 days.

blue fried rice with salmon

SERVINGS: 4
PREP TIME: 10 MIN
COOK TIME: 50 MIN

DAIRY-FREE
GLUTEN-FREE
(VEGAN OPTION)

superfoods used

SPIRULINA POWDER
SESAME OIL
GARLIC
CARROT
CELERY
GINGER
LIME
SESAME SEED
SALMON
BLUE BUTTERFLY PEA
POWDER

nutrition info

CALORIES: 397
FAT: 13
CARBS: 43
NET CARBS: 39
FIBER: 4
PROTEIN: 26

nutrition info for
vegan option

CALORIES: 395
FAT: 15
CARBS: 44
NET CARBS: 40
FIBER: 4
PROTEIN: 19

Spirulina is a great source of vitamins E, C, and B6. It's often added to sweet recipes, but it is wonderful in savory preparations such as this fried rice. Spirulina is an excellent source of plant-based protein and very nutrient dense. It has the ability to enhance our microbiome with its ability to boost IgA production. The blue butterfly pea powder is a great source of antioxidants and anthocyanins. For added protein and healthy fats, stir in a large egg and scramble into everything when you add the rice. Not only is this recipe beautiful, but it's also delicious!

BLUE FRIED RICE

- 1 cup (200 g) brown rice
- 2 cups (480 ml) water
- 1 teaspoon (3 g) spirulina powder
- 1 teaspoon (4 g) blue butterfly pea powder

VEGETABLES

- 1 tablespoon (15 ml) sesame oil
- 4 small (16 g) cloves garlic, minced
- 1 medium (80 g) carrot, peeled and shredded
- 1 cup (100 g) diced celery
- 1 tablespoon (6 g) peeled and grated fresh ginger
- 1 teaspoon (6 g) sea salt
- ½ teaspoon (3 g) black pepper
- 1 teaspoon (3 g) dried red pepper flakes
- ¼ cup (4 g) fresh cilantro, minced
- 1 medium (15 g) scallion, minced
- 1 tablespoon (10 g) black or white sesame seeds

SALMON

- 2 tablespoons (30 ml) sesame oil, divided
- 2 tablespoons (30 ml) coconut aminos
- 1 teaspoon (6 g) sea salt
- Zest from ½ medium (11 g) fresh lime
- 2 tablespoons (30 ml) fresh lime juice
- 1 pound (454 g) wild-caught salmon fillets (or 1 pound [454 g] extra-firm tofu, cubed)

To make the blue fried rice, rinse the rice well in a fine-mesh strainer. Add it with the water to a large pot on the stove. Cover and bring to a boil. Once boiling, decrease the heat to a simmer and cook until soft and fluffy, 40 to 45 minutes. When it is done, remove from the heat. Stir in the spirulina and blue butterfly pea powders until evenly combined and the rice is blue.

While the rice is cooking, prepare the vegetables and salmon. To make the vegetables, add the sesame oil to a large skillet over medium-high heat. Add the garlic, carrot, celery, ginger, salt, pepper, and red pepper flakes. Sauté until the vegetables are soft, about 5 minutes.

Add the blue rice to the skillet and continue to cook until the rice has absorbed the liquid from the vegetables. Stir in the cilantro, scallion, and sesame seeds. Transfer the rice to a serving bowl.

To make the salmon (or tofu), add 1 tablespoon (15 ml) of the sesame oil, coconut aminos, salt, and lime zest and juice to a small bowl. Whisk to combine. Brush the fillets (or tofu) with the sesame oil mixture.

Add the remaining 1 tablespoon (15 ml) sesame oil to the same skillet over medium-high heat. Place the salmon fillets (or tofu) in the skillet, skin-side down, not moving once in the skillet. Sear for 3 to 4 minutes per side, or until its flesh is opaque in color (or the tofu is golden). Turn off the heat.

Serve the salmon (or tofu) over the blue fried rice. Store any leftovers in the fridge in an airtight container for up to 2 days.

roasted plum chicken with quinoa and green beans

SERVINGS: 4
PREP TIME: 10 MIN PLUS
SOAKING OVERNIGHT
COOK TIME: 50 MIN

DAIRY-FREE
GLUTEN-FREE
GRAIN-FREE
(VEGAN OPTION)

superfoods used

**AVOCADO OIL
LEMON
CINNAMON
RED ONION
PLUM
QUINOA
THYME**

nutrition info

**CALORIES: 555
FAT: 29
CARBS: 45
NET CARBS: 37
FIBER: 8
PROTEIN: 28**

*nutrition info for
vegan option*

**CALORIES: 440
FAT: 17
CARBS: 46
NET CARBS: 38
FIBER: 8
PROTEIN: 25**

Adding fresh lemon slices to roast chicken (or tofu) creates caramelized bites of lemon and tender and delicious pieces of meat or vegan protein. Lemons are high in fiber and vitamin C. We don't typically consume plums in a hot meal with chicken, but the addition to this recipe gives it the antioxidant and anti-inflammatory boost it needs. These flavors work so well together and burst in your mouth, and they also work together in your gut to boost your microflora and digestive health.

PLUMS AND CHICKEN

- ¼ cup (60 ml) avocado oil
- 2 tablespoons (30 ml) fresh lemon juice
- 2 tablespoon (30 ml) balsamic vinegar
- 2 teaspoons (12 g) sea salt
- 1 teaspoon (6 g) black pepper
- 1 teaspoon (3 g) ground cinnamon
- Pinch of ground nutmeg
- 1 medium (150 g) red onion, sliced
- 4 medium (264 g) plums, pitted and sliced
- 1 medium (26 g) fresh lemon, sliced and seeds removed
- 1 pound (454 g) bone-in chicken thighs (or 1 pound [454 g] extra-firm tofu, sliced)

Preheat the oven to 400°F (200°C).

To make the plums and chicken, add the oil, lemon juice, balsamic vinegar, salt, pepper, cinnamon, and nutmeg to a large mixing bowl. Whisk well. Add the onion, plums, lemon, and chicken thighs (or tofu) to the bowl. Gently toss until everything is coated.

Arrange chicken (or tofu) and plums in a large, cast-iron skillet. Place the lemon slices on top of each chicken thigh (or tofu slice). Bake in the oven for 40 to 45 minutes, or until the chicken has reached 165°F (74°C). The onion, plums, and lemon slices will be soft and caramelized.

While the plums and chicken are cooking, prepare the quinoa. Rinse the soaked quinoa very well using a fine-mesh strainer, then transfer to a saucepan. Add the boiling water over low heat. Let the quinoa soak in the boiling water for about 10 minutes, or until it has soaked up all the water.

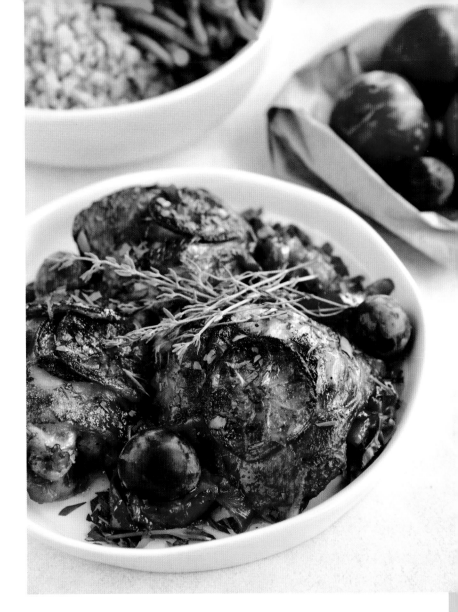

QUINOA

1 cup (200 g) quinoa
(soaked overnight in cold
water)

1¼ cups (300 ml) boiling
water

GREEN BEANS

1 pound (454 g) green
beans, ends trimmed

GARNISH

¼ cup (4 g) fresh parsley,
minced

Fresh thyme sprigs

To make the green beans, add 2 inches (5 cm)
of water to a medium pot on the stove over high
heat. Add the green beans to a steam basket
and steam until soft, 5 to 7 minutes. Set aside.

Remove the plums and chicken (or tofu) from
the oven. Garnish with the parsley and thyme.
Serve with the quinoa and green beans.
Store any leftovers in the fridge in an airtight
container for up to 3 days.

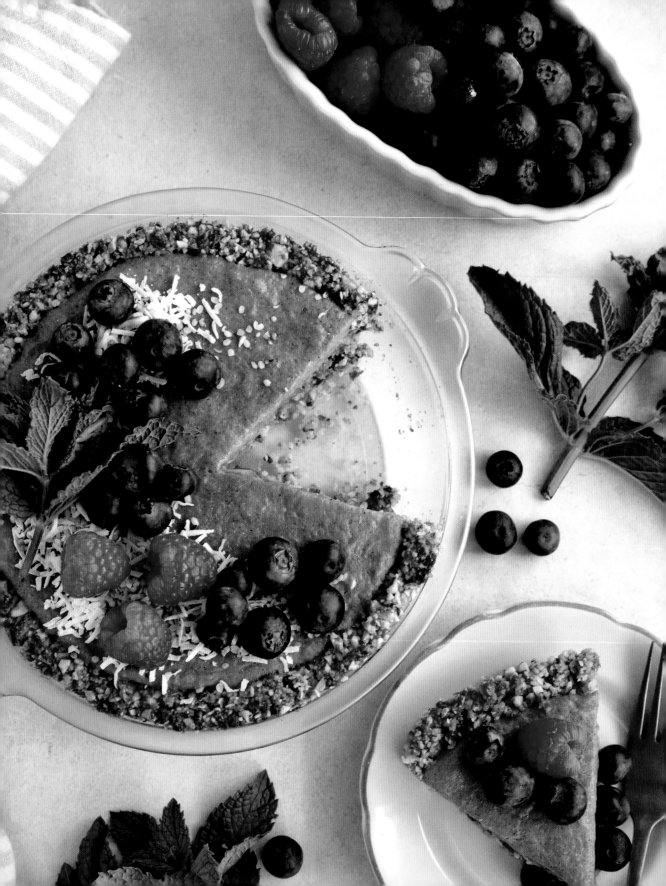

CHAPTER TEN

DESSERTS & TREATS

Desserts don't need to be high in processed sugars to be enjoyable. Try out these anti-inflammatory and nutrient-dense desserts for a satisfying treat. You will find a plethora of nuts, seeds, cacao, fruits, and even tahini (sesame paste) to make these decadent desserts. And you won't see inflammatory cane sugar in any of these recipes; instead, we'll sweeten things up with figs, dates, and maple syrup.

Can you picture a dessert with the anti-inflammatory superfood turmeric? Well, you will find it here! How about Tahini Chocolate Chip Cookies (page 183)? I bet you wouldn't think they would be part of the immunity food fix. The Fig and Apricot Almond Balls (page 175) are the perfect after meal sweet bite or even a midday, low-calorie snack. The Chocolate-Almond and Rose Cups (page 176) include several hidden ingredients that give it anti-inflammatory and antioxidant benefits—yet still a chocolate cup!

With the right ingredients you can create anything. So many superfoods can be hidden in the batter to give that anti-inflammatory, antioxidant, and immune-modulating boost. At your next gathering, wow your friends and family with one of these treats and the immunity-boosting ingredients you used to create them!

Pineapple Tart, page 180

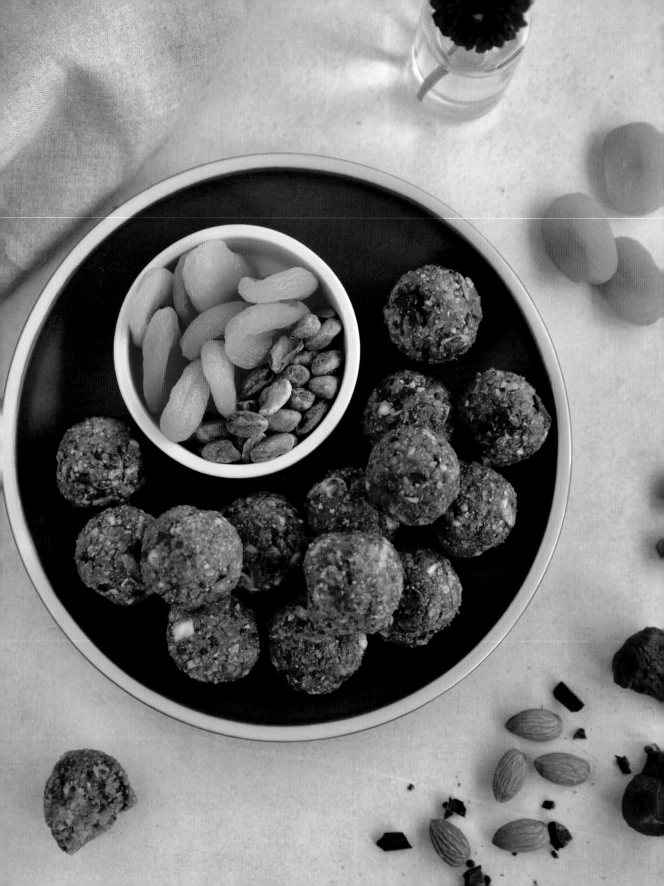

fig and apricot almond balls

Figs contain a polysaccharide that gives them their great antioxidant potential. Apricots, with their bright orange color, are plentiful in antioxidants and a great source of vitamin A. The nuts give this recipe good fatty acids, with a delicious combination of flavors! This treat is filled with vitamins A, E, C, and K as well as potassium, calcium, and iron. Plus, it is rich in beta-carotene and antioxidants! It's perfect as a dessert or even an on-the-go snack!

SERVINGS: 12
PREP TIME: 10 MIN
COOK TIME: 35 MIN

VEGAN
VEGETARIAN
DAIRY-FREE
GLUTEN-FREE
GRAIN-FREE

superfoods used

FIG
APRICOT
ALMOND
PISTACHIO
CINNAMON

nutrition info

CALORIES: 83
FAT: 4
CARBS: 10
NET CARBS: 8
FIBER: 2
PROTEIN: 2

BALLS

- 1 cup (150 g) dried figs, stems removed
- 1 cup (190 g) dried apricots, chopped
- 1 cup (143 g) raw almonds
- ½ cup (63 g) raw pistachios
- Pinch of sea salt
- 1 teaspoon (3 g) ground cinnamon
- 1 teaspoon (4 g) vanilla bean powder
- 3 tablespoons (21 g) cacao nibs

To make the balls, cover the dried figs and apricots with hot water. Let sit for 10 minutes.

Meanwhile, pulse the almonds and pistachios in a food processor until fine and crumbly. Add the salt, cinnamon, and vanilla bean powder. Pulse until well combined.

Drain the dried fruit and add it to the food processor, pulsing until everything is well combined and a "dough" has formed. Stir in the cacao nibs.

Using a tablespoon (15 g) measuring spoon, scoop a spoonful of the dough and roll it into a ball with your hands. Continue until you have used all of the dough (you should get about twelve balls).

Store any leftovers in the fridge in an airtight container for up to 2 weeks or the freezer for up to 3 months.

chocolate-almond and rose cups

SERVINGS: 12
PREP TIME: 5 MIN
COOK TIME: 10 MIN
PLUS 2 HOURS
TO CHILL

VEGAN
VEGETARIAN
DAIRY-FREE
GLUTEN-FREE
GRAIN-FREE

These chocolate cups are loaded with nutrients found in cacao, beet root powder, dates, and more. Cacao is unique because the procyanidins serve as a prebiotic, with the ability to increase good gut bacteria. Beet root powder is great for reducing inflammation and boosting antioxidants. Dates are an excellent source of fiber, and they also serve as a great natural sweetener in this recipe! The cups are delicious, and they contain healthy fats that help keep your blood sugar stable.

superfoods used

ALMOND
CINNAMON
BEET

nutrition info

CALORIES: 229
FAT: 16
CARBS: 23
NET CARBS: 19
FIBER: 4
PROTEIN: 5

CHOCOLATE CUPS

- 9 ounces (270 g) dark chocolate chips
- ½ cup (128 g) raw almond butter
- 1 teaspoon (3 g) ground cinnamon
- 1 teaspoon (4 g) vanilla bean powder
- 1 tablespoon (7.6 g) dried beet powder
- ½ cup (72 g) raw almonds, chopped
- 6 Medjool dates, pitted and chopped
- 2 tablespoons (6 g) dried culinary-grade rosebuds, chopped
- Sprinkle of sea salt

To make the cups, line a 12-cup muffin tin with silicone or parchment paper liners.

Add the chocolate chips to a small glass bowl and set it on top of a small saucepan filled with 2 cups (480 ml) of water. Bring to a simmer on the stove. Once simmering, stir often until the chocolate is melted. Turn off the heat and carefully remove the bowl from the saucepan.

Stir in the almond butter, cinnamon, vanilla bean powder, beet powder, almonds, and dates. Pour equal amounts into the muffin tin, and gently top each with the dried rosebuds and a sprinkle of salt. Place in the fridge to chill for 2 hours.

Serve and enjoy! Store any leftovers in the fridge in an airtight container for up to 2 weeks or the freezer for up to 3 months.

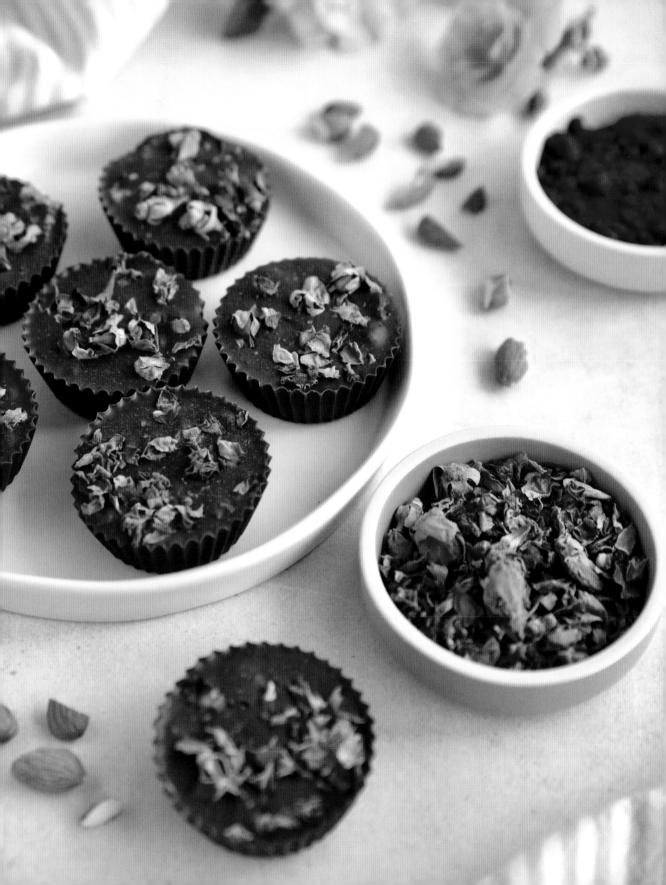

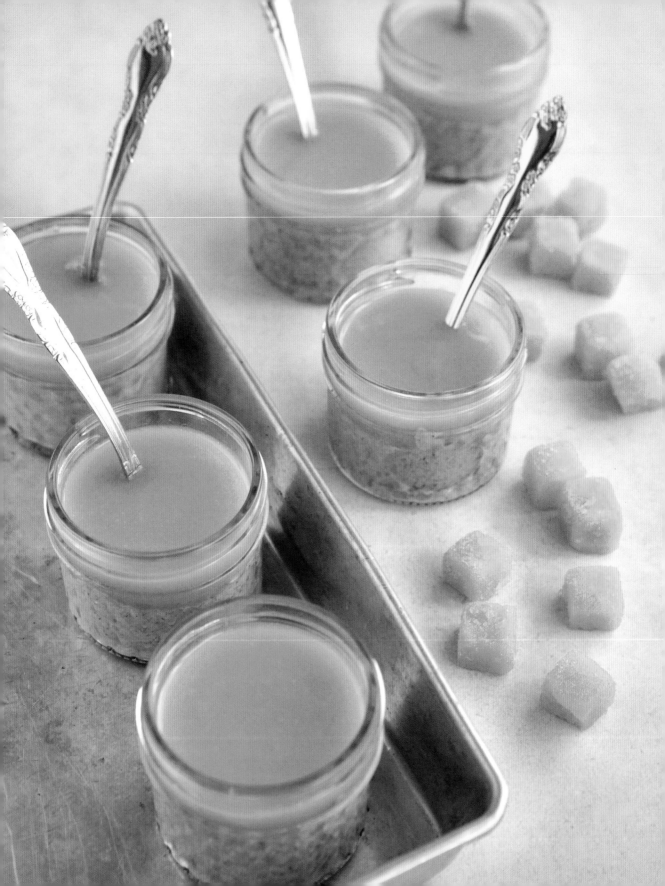

passion fruit panna cotta

Passion fruit is rich in iron, helping you to absorb vitamin C. It aids in digestion and increases immunity. They are smaller fruits, and you will need several fresh passion fruits to obtain a full cup of its pulp for this recipe. Opt to purchase the pulp only, which can be found in the freezer aisle at your market. The combination with almonds gives you added protein, fiber, and an antioxidant boost with its high vitamin E content. All this—in a dessert!

SERVINGS: 6
PREP TIME: 5 MIN
COOK TIME: 10 MIN
PLUS 4 HOURS
TO CHILL

DAIRY-FREE
GLUTEN-FREE
GRAIN-FREE
VEGAN

superfoods used

ALMOND
PASSION FRUIT

PANNA COTTA

- 1 cup (240 ml) plain, unsweetened almond milk or your choice of plant-based milk
- 1 cup (240 g) coconut cream
- 1 tablespoon (7 g) agar-agar powder
- 3 tablespoons (45 ml) maple syrup
- 2 teaspoons (8 g) vanilla bean powder
- 1 cup (200 g) passion fruit pulp

To make the panna cotta, add the almond milk and coconut cream to a saucepan over medium heat. Bring to a boil. Once boiling, decrease the heat to a simmer and stir in the agar-agar, maple syrup, and vanilla bean powder. Stir often for 3 minutes, then turn off the heat.

Pour into six small jars, leaving 2 to 3 inches (5 to 7.5 cm) of room at the top to fill with passion fruit pulp later. Transfer the jars to the fridge and completely chill, about 4 hours, before topping with the passion fruit pulp.

Serve and enjoy! Store any leftovers in the fridge in an airtight container for up to 5 days.

nutrition info

CALORIES: 155
FAT: 9
CARBS: 16
NET CARBS: 15
FIBER: 1
PROTEIN: 1

pineapple tart

SERVINGS: 8
PREP TIME: 20 MIN
COOK TIME: 10 MIN
PLUS 4 HOURS
TO CHILL

VEGETARIAN
VEGAN
DAIRY-FREE
GLUTEN-FREE
GRAIN-FREE

superfoods used

ALMOND
MACADAMIA NUT
PINEAPPLE
LIME
TURMERIC
BERRIES
PEPPERMINT
HEMP SEED

nutrition info

CALORIES: 444
FAT: 30
CARBS: 26
NET CARBS: 19
FIBER: 7
PROTEIN: 6

Pineapple is wonderful for improved digestion, and it is high in vitamin C, manganese, and fiber. Combining pineapple and coconut takes the flavors to the next level! You will find a hidden touch of turmeric, known for its anti-inflammatory properties. Macadamia nuts contain the highest amount of MUFAs and are excellent for reducing inflammation. Don't skip out on the garnish of berries and hemp seeds. They give you that added fiber and protein. Let this recipe transport you to the tropics with every naturally sweet bite!

CRUST

- 1 cup (143 g) raw almonds
- 1 cup (125 g) raw macadamia nuts
- ¾ cup (54 g) shredded unsweetened coconut
- ½ cup (112 g) dried dates, pitted
- 2 tablespoons (30 ml) avocado oil
- 1 tablespoon (15 ml) maple syrup
- Pinch of sea salt

FILLING

- 1 cup (240 g) coconut cream
- 2 cups (330 g) chopped fresh pineapple
- 3 tablespoons (45 ml) fresh lime juice
- 3 tablespoons (45 ml) maple syrup
- 2 teaspoons (8 g) vanilla bean powder
- ⅛ teaspoon ground turmeric
- 1 tablespoon (7 g) agar-agar powder

GARNISH

- ¼ cup (36 g) fresh berries
- 2 tablespoons (9 g) shredded unsweetened coconut
- 1 tablespoon (10 g) hemp seeds
- Fresh mint leaves, minced

Preheat the oven to 350°F (175°C). Line an 8-inch (20-cm) tart pan with parchment paper.

To make the crust, pulse the ingredients in a food processor until fine and crumbly, scraping down the sides of the bowl as needed. Using your hands, press it firmly into the bottom of the prepared tart pan and up the sides, creating a crust. Bake in the oven for 10 minutes, then remove and let cool.

While the crust is baking, prepare the filling. Add all the ingredients except the agar-agar powder to a high-speed blender. Pulse until very creamy. Transfer to a saucepan on the stove and bring to a simmer. Once simmering, add the agar-agar powder and whisk well to combine.

Pour the pineapple filling into the cooled crust, transfer to the fridge, and completely chill, about 4 hours.

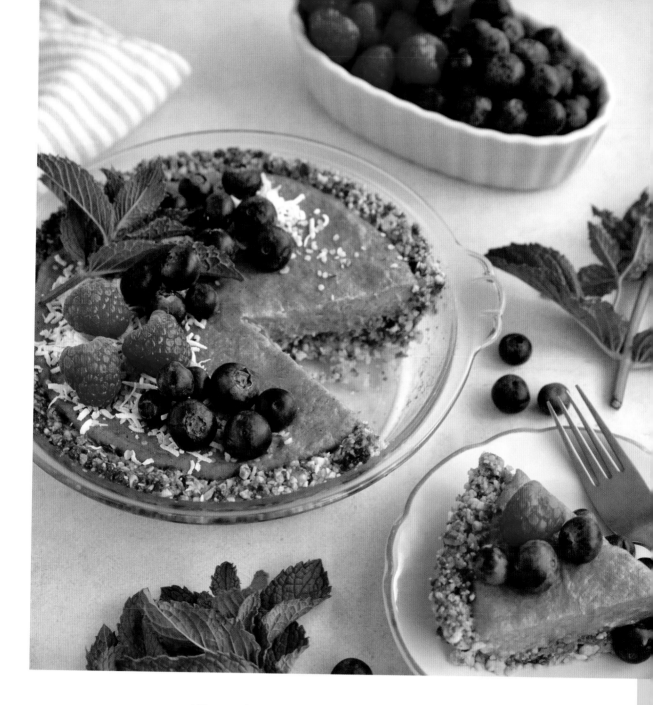

When cool, garnish with the berries, shredded coconut, hemp seeds, and mint.

Serve and enjoy! Store any leftovers in the fridge in an airtight container for up to 5 days.

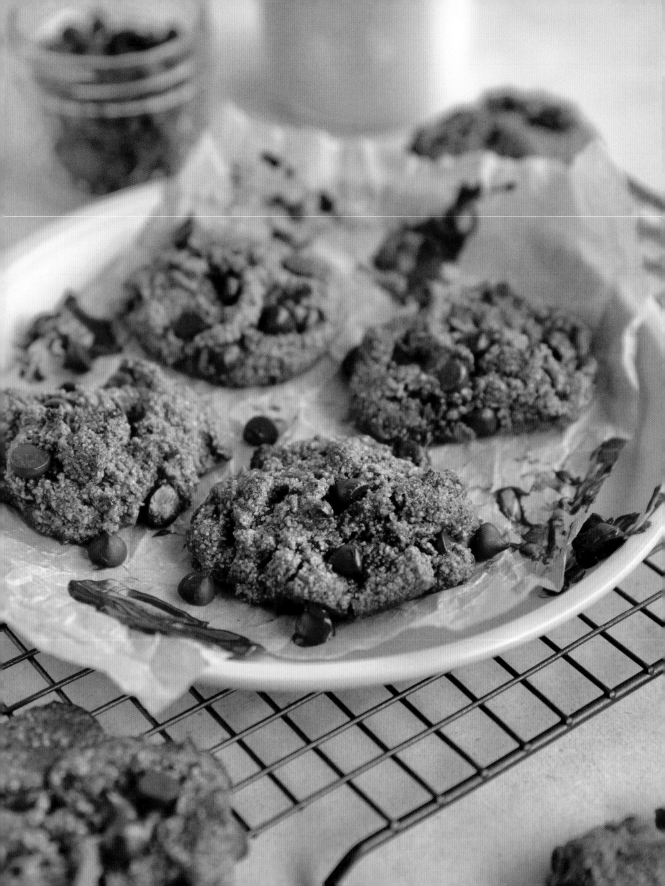

tahini chocolate chip cookies

The combination of almond flour, creamy tahini, and a hint of maple syrup creates the most delicious caramel flavor and a delicately crunchy texture. The flax meal as an egg alternative in this recipe helps create balance in our gut bacteria, adding great omega-3 content and being anti-inflammatory in nature. These cookies are high in magnesium among other vitamins and nutrients that support your immune system, and they are sure to become a staple in your kitchen!

MAKES: 12 COOKIES (SERVING SIZE IS 1 COOKIE)
PREP TIME: 10 MIN
COOK TIME: 10 MIN

VEGAN
DAIRY-FREE
GLUTEN-FREE
GRAIN-FREE

superfoods used

ALMOND
FLAXSEED
CINNAMON
SESAME SEED
AVOCADO OIL

COOKIES

- 2 teaspoons (4 g) flax meal
- 2 tablespoons (30 ml) water
- 1 cup (100 g) almond flour
- ½ teaspoon (3 g) sea salt
- 1 teaspoon (3 g) ground cinnamon
- 1 teaspoon (4 g) vanilla bean powder
- ½ teaspoon (2 g) baking powder
- 2 tablespoons (30 g) tahini
- 2 teaspoons (10 ml) avocado oil
- ¼ cup (60 g) maple syrup
- ¼ cup (85 g) dark chocolate chips

Preheat the oven to 375°F (190°C). Line a baking sheet with parchment paper.

To make the cookies, mix the flax and water in a small bowl. Let it thicken for 5 minutes.

Mix the almond flour, salt, cinnamon, vanilla bean powder, and baking powder in a mixing bowl. In a separate bowl, mix the tahini, oil, and maple syrup.

Add the tahini mixture and the flax mixture to the dry ingredients and gently mix until a dough has formed and there are no dry spots. Gently fold in the chocolate chips.

Form 2-inch (5-cm) balls of dough with your hands and gently flatten before arranging on the prepared baking sheet. Bake for 7 to 10 minutes, checking to ensure they do not burn.

When golden in color, remove from the oven, then lift the parchment paper up and set it on a cooling rack to prevent the hot pan from further cooking the cookies. Let cool for 2 to 3 minutes.

Serve and enjoy! Store any leftovers in an airtight container for up to 3 days or the freezer for up to 3 months.

nutrition info

CALORIES: 111
FAT: 7
CARBS: 9
NET CARBS: 7
FIBER: 2
PROTEIN: 3

REFERENCES

CHAPTER ONE

Achamrah, Najate, Pierre Déchelotte, and Moïse Coëffier. "Glutamine and the Regulation of Intestinal Permeability: From Bench to Bedside." *Current Opinion in Clinical Nutrition & Metabolic Care* 20, no. 1 (2017): 86–91.

Barbuzano, Javier. "Understanding How the Intestine Replaces and Repairs Itself." *The Harvard Gazette* July 14, 2017.

Burr, Ansen H. P., Amrita Bhattacharjee, and Timothy W. Hand. "Nutritional Modulation of the Microbiome and Immune Response." *The Journal of Immunology* 205, no. 6 (2020): 1479–1487.

Childs, Caroline E., Philip C. Calder, and Elizabeth A. Miles. "Diet and Immune Function." *Nutrients* 11, no. 8 (2019): 1–9.

Duboc, H., D. Rainteau, S. Rajca, L. Humbert, D. Farabos, M. Maubert, V. Grondin, et al. "Increase in Fecal Primary Bile Acids and Dysbiosis in Patients with Diarrhea-Predominant Irritable Bowel Syndrome." *Neurogastroenterology & Motility* 24, no. 6 (2012): 513-520.

Duboc, Henri, Sylvie Rajca, Dominique Rainteau, David Benarous, Marie-Anne Maubert, Elodie Quervain, Ginette Thomas, et al. "Connecting Dysbiosis, Bile Acid Dysmetabolism and Gut Inflammation in Inflammatory Bowel Diseases." *Gut* 62, no. 4 (2013): 531–539.

Gummesson, Anders, Lena M. S. Carlsson, Len H. Storlien, Fredrik Bäckhed, Pål Lundin, Lars Löfgren, Kaj Stenlöf, Yan Y. Lam, Björn Fagerberg, and Björn Carlsson. "Intestinal Permeability Is Associated with Visceral Adiposity in Healthy Women." *Obesity* 19, no. 11 (2011): 2280–2282.

Harvey, Natasha L. "The Link between Lymphatic Function and Adipose Biology." *Annals of the New York Academy of Sciences* 1131, no. 1 (2008): 82–88.

Hollon, Justin, Elaine Leonard Puppa, Bruce Greenwald, Eric Goldberg, Anthony Guerrerio, and Alessio Fasano. "Effect of Gliadin on Permeability of Intestinal Biopsy Explants from Celiac Disease Patients and Patients with Non-Celiac Gluten Sensitivity." *Nutrients* 7, no. 3 (2015): 1565–1576.

Lammers, Karen M., Ruliang Lu, Julie Brownley, Bao Lu, Craig Gerard, Karen Thomas, Prasad Rallabhandi, et al. "Gliadin Induces an Increase in Intestinal Permeability and Zonulin Release by Binding to the Chemokine Receptor CXCR3." *Gastroenterology* 135, no. 1 (2008): 194–204.

Shi, Na, Na Li, Xinwang Duan, and Haitao Niu. "Interaction between the Gut Microbiome and Mucosal Immune System." *Military Medical Research* 4, no. 1 (2017): 1–7.

Suzuki, Takuya, and Hiroshi Hara. "Dietary Fat and Bile Juice, but Not Obesity, Are Responsible for the Increase in Small Intestinal Permeability Induced through the Suppression of Tight Junction Protein Expression in LETO and OLETF Rats." *Nutrition & Metabolism* 7, no. 1 (2010): 1–17.

Tran, Cuong D., Desma M. Grice, Ben Wade, Caroline A. Kerr, Denis C. Bauer, Dongmei Li, and Garry N. Hannan. "Gut Permeability, Its Interaction with Gut Microflora and Effects on Metabolic Health Are Mediated by the Lymphatics System, Liver and Bile Acid." *Future Microbiology* 10, no. 8 (2015): 1339–1353.

CHAPTER TWO

Akramienė, Dalia, Anatolijus Kondrotas, Janina Didžiapetrienė, and Egidijus Kėvelaitis. "Effects of ß-glucans on the Immune System." *Medicina* 43, no. 8 (2007): 597–606.

Al-Khalaifah, Hanan. "Modulatory Effect of Dietary Polyunsaturated Fatty Acids on Immunity, Represented by Phagocytic Activity." *Frontiers in Veterinary Science* 7 (2020): 1-11.

Calder, Philip C., Anitra C. Carr, Adrian F. Gombart, and Manfred Eggersdorfer. "Optimal Nutritional Status for a Well-Functioning Immune System Is an Important Factor to Protect against Viral Infections." *Nutrients* 12, no. 4 (2020): 1-6.

Cruzat, Vinicius, Marcelo Macedo Rogero, Kevin Noel Keane, Rui Curi, and Philip Newsholme. "Glutamine: Metabolism and Immune Function, Supplementation and Clinical Translation." *Nutrients* 10, no. 11 (2018): 1-21.

Daly, John M., John Reynolds, Robert K. Sigal, J. I. A. N. Shou, and Michael D. Liberman. "Effect of Dietary Protein and Amino Acids on Immune Function." *Critical Care Medicine* 18, no. 2 Suppl (1990): S86–93.

De Souza Breda, Cristiane Naffah, Gustavo Gastão Davanzo, Paulo José Basso, Niels Olsen Saraiva Câmara, and Pedro Manoel Mendes Moraes-Vieira. "Mitochondria as Central Hub of the Immune System." *Redox Biology* 26 (2019): 1-12.

Elmadfa, Ibrahim, and Alexa L. Meyer. "The Role of the Status of Selected Micronutrients in Shaping the Immune Function." *Endocrine, Metabolic & Immune Disorders-Drug Targets* 19, no. 8 (2019): 1100–1115.

Faas, M. M., and P. De Vos. "Mitochondrial Function in Immune Cells in Health and Disease." *Biochimica et Biophysica Acta (BBA)-Molecular Basis of Disease* 1866, no. 10 (2020): 1-9.

Gombart, Adrian F., Adeline Pierre, and Silvia Maggini. "A Review of Micronutrients and the Immune System—Working in Harmony to Reduce the Risk of Infection." *Nutrients* 12, no. 1 (2020): 1-31.

Li, Peng, Yu-Long Yin, Defa Li, Sung Woo Kim, and Guoyao Wu. "Amino Acids and Immune Function." *British Journal of Nutrition* 98, no. 2 (2007): 237–252.

Martin-Gallausiaux, Camille, Ludovica Marinelli, Hervé M. Blottière, Pierre Larraufie, and Nicolas Lapaque. "SCFA: Mechanisms and Functional Importance in the Gut." *Proceedings of the Nutrition Society* 80, no. 1 (2021): 37–49.

Radzikowska, Urszula, Arturo O. Rinaldi, Zeynep Çelebi Sözener, Dilara Karaguzel, Marzena Wojcik, Katarzyna Cypryk, Mübeccel Akdis, Cezmi A. Akdis, and Milena Sokolowska. "The Influence of Dietary Fatty Acids on Immune Responses." *Nutrients* 11, no. 12 (2019): 1-32.

Shokryazdan, Parisa, Mohammad Faseleh Jahromi, Bahman Navidshad, and Juan Boo Liang. "Effects of Prebiotics on Immune System and Cytokine Expression." *Medical Microbiology and Immunology* 206, no. 1 (2017): 1–9.

Tourkochristou, Evanthia, Christos Triantos, and Athanasia Mouzaki. "The Influence of Nutritional Factors on Immunological Outcomes." *Frontiers in Immunology* 12 (2021): 1-12.

Walker, Melissa A., Stefano Volpi, Katherine B. Sims, Jolan E. Walter, and Elisabetta Traggiai. "Powering the Immune System: Mitochondria in Immune Function and Deficiency." *Journal of Immunology Research* 2014 (2014): 1-6.

Wastyk, Hannah C., Gabriela K. Fragiadakis, Dalia

Perelman, Dylan Dahan, Bryan D. Merrill, B. Yu Feiqiao, Madeline Topf, et al. "Gut-Microbiota-Targeted Diets Modulate Human Immune Status." *Cell* 184, no. 16 (2021): 4137–4153.

CHAPTER THREE

Chapman, Nicole M., and Hongbo Chi. "Metabolic Adaptation of Lymphocytes in Immunity and Disease." *Immunity* 55, no. 1 (2022): 14–30.

Fong, Ted Chun Tat. "Indirect Effects of Body Mass Index Growth on Glucose Dysregulation via Inflammation: Causal Moderated Mediation Analysis." *Obesity Facts* 12, no. 3 (2019): 316–327.

Goodpaster, Bret H., and Lauren M. Sparks. "Metabolic Flexibility in Health and Disease." *Cell Metabolism* 25, no. 5 (2017): 1-11.

Kalupahana, Nishan S., Naima Moustaid-Moussa, and Kate J. Claycombe. "Immunity as a Link between Obesity and Insulin Resistance." *Molecular Aspects of Medicine* 33, no. 1 (2012): 26–34.

Khan, Shahanshah, Sumyya Waliullah, Victoria Godfrey, Abdul Wadud Khan, Rajalaksmy A. Ramachandran, Brandi L. Cantarel, Cassie Behrendt, Lan Peng, Lora V. Hooper, and Hasan Zaki. "Dietary Simple Sugars Alter Microbial Ecology in the Gut and Promote Colitis in Mice." *Science Translational Medicine* 12, no. 567 (2020): 1-14.

Lee, Yun Sok, and Jerrold Olefsky. "Chronic Tissue Inflammation and Metabolic Disease." *Genes & Development* 35, no. 5–6 (2021): 307–328.

Lee, Yun Sok, Joshua Wollam, and Jerrold M. Olefsky. "An Integrated View of Immunometabolism." *Cell* 172, no. 1–2 (2018): 1-21.

Olefsky, Jerrold M., and Christopher K. Glass. "Macrophages, Inflammation, and Insulin Resistance." *Annual Review of Physiology* 72 (2010): 219–246.

Winer, Daniel A., Helen Luck, Sue Tsai, and Shawn Winer. "The Intestinal Immune System in Obesity and Insulin Resistance." *Cell Metabolism* 23, no. 3 (2016): 413–426.

CHAPTER FOUR

Cline, John C. "Nutritional Aspects of Detoxification in Clinical Practice." *Alternative Therapies in Health & Medicine* 21, no. 3 (2015): 54–62.

Fowke, Jay H., Jason D. Morrow, Saundra Motley, Roberd M. Bostick, and Reid M. Ness. "Brassica Vegetable Consumption Reduces Urinary F2-isoprostane Levels Independent of Micronutrient Intake." *Carcinogenesis* 27, no. 10 (2006): 2096–2102.

Fukao, T., T. Hosono, S. Misawa, T. Seki, and T. Ariga. "The Effects of Allyl Sulfides on the Induction of Phase II Detoxification Enzymes and Liver Injury by Carbon Tetrachloride." *Food and Chemical Toxicology* 42, no. 5 (2004): 743–749.

Jancova, Petra, Pavel Anzenbacher, and Eva Anzenbacherova. "Phase II Drug Metabolizing Enzymes." *Biomedical Papers of the Medical Faculty of the University Palacky, Olomouc, Czechoslovakia* 154, no. 2 (2010): 103–116.

Jovanovski, Elena, Shahen Yashpal, Allison Komishon, Andreea Zurbau, Sonia Blanco Mejia, Hoang Vi Thanh Ho, Dandan Li, John Sievenpiper, Lea Duvnjak, and Vladimir Vuksan. "Effect of Psyllium (*Plantago ovata*) Fiber on LDL Cholesterol and Alternative Lipid Targets, Non-HDL Cholesterol and Apolipoprotein B:

A Systematic Review and Meta-Analysis of Randomized Controlled Trials." *The American Journal of Clinical Nutrition* 108, no. 5 (2018): 922–932.

Liska, DeAnn J., and Jeffrey S. Bland. "Emerging Clinical Science of Bifunctional Support for Detoxification." *Townsend Letter for Doctors and Patients* 231 (2002): 42–47.

Liston, Heidi L., John S. Markowitz, and C. Lindsay DeVane. "Drug Glucuronidation in Clinical Psychopharmacology." *Journal of Clinical Psychopharmacology* 21, no. 5 (2001): 500–515.

Odenthal, Julia, Björn W. H. van Heumen, Hennie M. J. Roelofs, Rene H. M. te Morsche, Brigitte Marian, Fokko M. Nagengast, and Wilbert H. M. Peters. "The Influence of Curcumin, Quercetin, and Eicosapentaenoic Acid on the Expression of Phase II Detoxification Enzymes in the Intestinal Cell Lines HT-29, Caco-2, HuTu 80, and LT97." *Nutrition and Cancer* 64, no. 6 (2012): 856–863.

Shenkin, A. "Micronutrients in Health and Disease." *Postgraduate Medical Journal* 82, no. 971 (2006): 559–567.

ACKNOWLEDGMENTS

Upon publishing *Immunity Food Fix*, I knew it was only the beginning of educating the world on the healing power of food. I have lived and breathed this lifestyle for more than eight years, and experimenting, learning, and applying all my knowledge to my everyday life and my family's. As a pharmacist, it's now become my purpose to bridge the gap between nutrition and medicine, between Eastern and Western medicine, and between conventional and functional medicine. There doesn't need to be a divide, and it's become my commitment to show the world the research and science on food is just as plentiful as the research and science on medicine, and we need both.

I thank my family for supporting me and following along as I implement my learnings in our lifestyle and for embracing every part of the journey. They are always troopers as I create new recipes and try new foods when I learn about their healing powers, without pushback or saying no. I'm proud of my girls, who have taken what I've taught them and spread it to their friends and teachers, helping to further educate the world.

I appreciate every follower on @drautoimmunegirl who has also spread the word and applied what I've taught them, and every message and outcome toward a better health brings me joy.

Thank you to Jill and the team at Fair Winds Press for continuing this opportunity to take the *Immunity Food Fix* to the next level and giving the world the applicability of everything they learned through this compilation of amazing recipes. Thank you to Sarah for your amazing recipe ideas and working together to make this dream a reality.

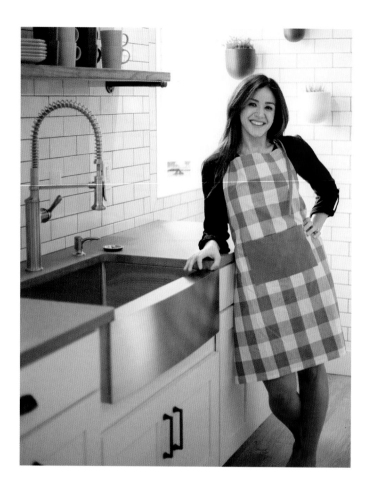

ABOUT THE AUTHOR

Donna Mazzola is the author of *Immunity Food Fix*, a science-backed guide on food as medicine and the research to support the benefits of plant-based foods. As a pharmacist, Donna had little education in nutrition and the impact of food on disease development and prevention. Through her own health struggles with autoimmunity, she furthered her education in human nutrition and functional medicine to bridge the gap between nutrition and medicine. After years of research, education, and personal experimentation, she learned the healing powers of food and applied them to her personal healing journey with autoimmunity. This led to the birth of DrAutoimmuneGirl, her persona and passion to empower people to take control of their health through diet and lifestyle interventions. The *Immunity Food Fix* is a compilation of all her knowledge and education to create the balance between nutrition and medicine. Follow her on Facebook, Pinterest, and Instagram @drautoimmunegirl

Photo by Nicolette Todor Photography

INDEX